A
NURSE'S
LEGACY

NOMATHEMBA MAZALENI

A
NURSE'S
LEGACY

LESSONS FROM A LIFE OF SERVICE

INSPiRED
PUBLISHING

A Nursey's Legacy: Lessons from A Life of Service
First Edition, First Impression 2021
ISBN: 978-1-77630-667-1
Copyright © Nomathemba Mazaleni

Published by:
Inspired Publishing
PO Box 82058 | Southdale | 2135
Johannesburg, South Africa Email: info@inspiredpublishing.co.za
www.inspiredpublishing.co.za

The stories in this book reflect the author's recollection of events. Some names, locations and identifying characteristics have been changed to protect the privacy of those depicted. Dialogue has been recreated from memory.

TABLE OF CONTENTS

ACKNOWLEDGEMENTS

I would like to thank my daughter, Pinky, and her husband, Fintan, who had confidence in me that I could write this book. They said it often enough so that I would actually start!

My brother, Mthuthuzeli Mabukane, helped me put together the family history and even showed me old, yellow-stained certificates which belonged to my elder sisters. Thank you Bra Mthura!

Thanks to Mandisa Mpotulo who nagged me, every time we met, about writing this book. She gave me the idea of referring to my passport stamps to document my travels in a chronological manner.

I am grateful to all the people I have worked with, in the different organisations, for some of the insights that I drew from them. The nurses whom I have trained and other professionals whom I have worked with and from whom I have learned a lot.

Lastly, I would like to thank Darren August from Inspired Publishing who really inspired me and made me believe that I could do it. Thanks, Darren for inspiring and holding my hand throughout the entire process.

DEDICATION

This book is dedicated to all the young girls and boys who come from humble backgrounds like me. Most importantly, to my sisters and brothers around the world - the NURSES. This book is meant to encourage them and that no matter where you started from, if you know where you are going, then life is a journey and you must enjoy the ride.

There are over 400 000 registered nurses in South Africa. Nurses play a central role in the health-care system of this country and in most countries around the world. We all have stories to tell. I am sharing mine in the hope that nurses of my age will relate to the stories. I also hope that young people in general, and young nurses in particular, will learn from it. I have been a nurse all my life and if I were to start my life all over again, I would still be a nurse.

This book outlines my travels, which I might have had trouble in remembering had it not been for all the stamps in my passports. I have five passports and I didn't hand in any of them when they expired. Some of the country stamps I see on my passports bring a smile to my face while others leave me asking a constant question which go something like:" What the hell was I doing in this place?"

My travels span over a period of 26 years and more than 50 cities, towns and villages on four continents. All the numerous trips I have undertaken were not paid for by me. Someone or another organisation paid for them. The fun, fear and lessons learned along the way should teach young nurses about the courage, leadership and resilience that our profession instils in us at an early age. This book shares the humble beginnings of a typical black women who is motivated and influenced by many to travel and see the world.

Many of the stories shared in this book will be familiar as they have been shared with nurses and other health workers in various meeting and workshops. In most cases the stories were meant to be therapeutic and to motivate them so that they would take up challenges and rise above their current situations.

This book is also dedicated to my grandchildren, Hope Mangaliso, Aidan Lizo and Connor Rolihlahla Hartnett. Written at the height of the coronavirus pandemic, it is significant as the pandemic has changed significant parts of our live - especially travel - which is the only way I can ever see my grandchildren again.

The world is watching an invisible virus killing thousands of people all over the world which affects us as we are part of the global village. It is defining the way we communicate and keep in touch with our loved ones. Relatives and grandmothers like me are left wondering when we will see our children and grandchildren who are on other continents and are equally affected by the pandemic. We are left with questions like "will I be able to hug my grandchildren again? Will they remember my face after all is said and done? They may remember the face, but what will they have to tell their own children about the maternal side of their lives?" These are scary thoughts and - depending on your mood – it may depress you. The lockdown is not helping at all.

It should make my grandchildren understand that with their Irish Canadian citizenship, they have African blood, which makes them citizens of all countries where there are black and white people. It should also make them understand that they should go out there and claim their world citizenship. The journey of their grandmother should remind them of their mixed origin and rich African roots which make them welcome in both parts of the world. Most of all, it should make them never to see colour in anybody and only see a human being.

The book also sheds light on their mother's life. May they never forget that it is a brave decision that she took to leave everything that she knows and the people who she loves, to settle in a foreign country to be with their father. To make sure that they grow up amongst their father's family and get used to a life that will be finally theirs. This book sheds a light on her upbringing as well as how their mother's bravery and travels shaped her and gave her the courage to leave South Africa.

Hopefully the pictures will wet their appetites and encourage them to follow in their grandmother's footsteps.

CHAPTER 1

MY FAMILY

I was born into the Mabukane family on the 22 June 1952. I was born in Hankey in the Gamtoos Valley, which is in the Sarah Baartman District of the Eastern Cape, Province of South Africa.

My father Ebenezer Lizo Mabukane was a warm and loving man who loved all his children and gave each one of us nicknames. I was his favourite and all my siblings knew this. He was a religious man and a leader in church. From him I learned the value of prayer.

My father, was a primary school teacher. He studied his teacher training qualifications at Healdtown High and Training College in Fort Beaufort. He used to boast that he was there at the time when our first democratically elected president, Nelson Rolihlahla Mandela, was also at the college.

My father taught in many schools in the province, including Greenbushes which is 58 km from his home in Hankey. He went as far as Cradock, which was 316 km away. My family moved from Hankey to Mdantsane in the early 1970s, where my father taught at Dickson Dyani Primary School. He later moved to Alice and taught at Gwali Primary School and eventually retired at the age of 70. He built the family home where I have retired in Krwakrwa Village in Alice.

My mother Singiswa Louisa Nobandla (born Kato) was a domestic worker who also worked in the Gamtoos Valley potato and tomato fields to support her husband. She was, like all mothers in this country, committed to educating her children and giving them the education that she never had. My mother did not know what grade each one of us was studying at a time. She was told by my father who was going to boarding school and she prepared accordingly. She was a loving and hard-working woman. From her, I learned the value of hard work.

In 1943 my parents were blessed with their first child, a daughter called Victoria Nomathamsanqa. They were very happy and excited but their joy was cut short as Nomathamsanqa died within two weeks.

In 1945, they were again blessed with a son named Mthuthuzeli Witness. Mthuthuzeli means "Comforter" and they felt that they were being comforted for the loss of their first child. Mthuthuzeli really became their comforter. He followed in my father's footsteps and studied in Healdtown High School. He later studied motor mechanics at Teko Vocational School in Butterworth. He is now 75 years old and my only surviving sibling.

Two years later, in 1947, they were blessed again with another daughter, Nozizwe Elizabeth. She also died two weeks after birth. The loss of their second daughter devastated them.

In 1950, they were blessed yet with another son. They named him Ntobeko. which means "Respect" or "Harmony". He survived. Ntobeko Hornabrook, the brother I come after, was the black sheep of the family when he was growing up. Many a time in Healdtown, he narrowly escaped expulsion. At one stage he was saved from expulsion by one of the teachers, who was also my father's former classmate at Healdtown – Mr Galaza Stamper.

Despite all his escapades, Ntobeko passed Matric and was admitted to the University of Fort Hare. He was the first - and only one of us - who managed to study at the famous 100-year-old institution, where the late President Nelson Mandela also studied. Ntobeko did not graduate from Fort Hare as he was later expelled for participating in the political uprisings of the 1970s. He eventually went into exile just after the death and burial of Steve Biko.

After months, we realised that Ntobeko had left to join the African National Congress (ANC) in exile, where he died. This we learned of through the newspapers and years later I managed to get a death certificate, that was written in Portuguese, from the ANC at Luthuli House. When we learnt that he died in Angola this helped to bring some closure to my family. The family could then hold a small memorial service in his honour.

On a cold winter's day, on 22 June 1952, Nobandla gave birth to a fragile and tiny baby girl. Everyone present was surprised at how small the baby was. My father's eldest sister, Nomangesi Matrose, was the midwife who delivered the baby. She asked for the baby's name and no one answered as they had not yet decided on the baby's name. According to my father, they had no hope that I would make it beyond the two weeks that my sisters had survived.

Ten days after I was born, my fathers' cousin - Themba (meaning Hope) Feni - came to visit. He was shocked that the baby still had no name. My parents told him that they had no hope that I was going to make it as I reminded them of the two girls that they had lost.

Uncle Themba told them to have Hope. He named me Nomathemba (meaning mother of Hope) after himself, because he had HOPE that I would live. This story that I heard when I asked why I was the only one without an English second name as all my siblings had English names. In the old apartheid days this was a problem when filling in forms or opening an account. Being served by a white person, I was always asked for my English name. I was followed by three siblings, all girls; Nokuthula Dora (nicknamed Thula), Koleka Christina (Connie) and Zoliswa Sarah (Nzoro). All born in 1955,1958 and 1961 respectively.

I started and finished my primary school at Centerton Public School in Hankey. From Standard three until Standard six, I was competing for the first position with one girl, Titi Mkonto. We both passed standard six with first class passes.

I proceeded to Healdtown High School, which was a most exciting time for me. I was counted amongst the naughty ones both in class and in the hostel, I got into all sorts of mischief with anybody. I just joined any group that was up to mischief.

At Healdtown's Girls Hostel we looked up to our prefects such as Nandipha Koyana, Timbela Ntlabati and many others. However, the best one was our chief prefect, Hazel Mangcu. Not only was she the most beautiful person that I had ever seen but she also carried herself so well and had such good command of English.

We, as the first-year students, would all fall quiet when she stood in front of us. We thought she was one of the wardens and only realised that she was a student when we saw her in the maroon and gold uniform. Maybe it was to control my mischief that I was made a prefect when I was in grade eleven. This did not stop me from getting up to all sorts of mischief, ranging from dodging church by sitting in the toilet, playing the piano during study time and talking after the lights out bell at night. Even though I was a prefect, I still got punished like everyone else.

I spent most of my primary and high school holidays in Walmer Township in Port Elizabeth staying with my uncle Nzima and aunt Nqabakazi Dlova. Coming from a middle-class family, by the standards of those days, I did not have many of the things that children from rich homes had. Most of my clothes were second hand that my mother got from the white ladies who she worked for.

My aunt Nqabakazi made up for this. Each holiday spent in Walmer meant that I would get new clothes. She would say: "I want you to look like all the children at the boarding school and in the neighbourhood." Her love and generosity were displayed in my last year during the matric farewell. She bought me the most beautiful dress, gold shoes and a matching handbag. She did all these things because she loved and felt sorry for her brother, my father, who was struggling to educate his six children.

The time spent with my uncle and aunt Nqabakazi taught me a lot. There were many of us who stayed in their home although they only had two children who were both grown up and married. They became mother and father to the children of relatives. They were running a small fruit and vegetables business and also sold meat. This meant I woke up as early as 5am to go help my aunt at the market.

It also meant that we had plenty of fruit, meat and vegetables to eat. Many people would buy on credit and promise to pay at the end of the week. My aunt knew the bad payers and, after resting from our trip to the market on Fridays, she would march us like her troop of solders to go and remind those who were supposed to come and pay. When they told my aunt stories of their husbands coming to pay after work, she would simply say to one of us: "Take the primus stove. They won't cook until they pay Nqabakazi's money."

In other houses she would tell us to take all blankets from the bed, which they would get when they paid their debt. One of my Aunt Nqabakazi's daughter, Pathiwe Qawu, was a nurse at Baragwanath Hospital in Johannesburg. She was beautiful, well dressed and we all admired and looked up to her. She inspired me to become a nurse.

I was in my last year at Healdtown when my sister joined me. She was fortunate to come to the school and join an elder sister who was there to protect her. Her joining me in the boarding school meant that my father had to pay for boarding, school fees and books for two children in Healdtown and my brother at the University of Fort Hare. My father prioritised Nokuthula boarding, school fees and books as she was new at the school. I was fortunate to get a bursary for my boarding fees which left my father with only the school fees and books to pay for.

This meant that I was the last one to get books in my class. Children being children, my classmates laughed when one of the teachers announced that I was the only one whose books had not yet been paid for. My response was typically the one I have used many a time. I told them: "You can all laugh, but I am going to be number one in this class, even without the books." And I was. I was competing for that position with people like Wallace Mgoqi, who is now an advocate in Cape Town, Mcebisi Mavuya and Fundiswa Mazwi.

Connie. who is younger than Nokuthula, went to Healdtown in 1973. They were fortunate that I was then a student nurse at Frere Hospital and earning some money. Knowing hostel life, I made sure that they did not want for anything that is needed in a boarding school.

Nzoro, the last born, is the only one who did not go to Healdtown as it burned down during riots. She did her secondary school education at Nyameko High School in Mdantsane and went to Themba Labantu High School in Zwelitsha where she matriculated.

We were very close as sisters and spent a lot of time together. Connie was the one with a deep sense of humour and always told stories that kept us in stiches. Sadly, all three of them have passed away. Left with my eldest brother, Mthuthuzeli, I decided to join him in the family home in Krwakrwa when I retired.

My father did well with his children as three of us qualified as nurses. Thula and Nzoro trained and qualified at Livingstone Hospital. Connie decided to follow in my father's footsteps and became a teacher. She did her teacher training at Rubusana Training College in Mdantsane.

I met and married my husband, Mncedisi Mazaleni, when I was working as a nurse at Frere Hospital. He was a high school teacher. We had one child Pinky Babalwa, which means "blessing".

I had grown up from a tiny and fragile baby and had developed into a young, vibrant and strong woman. Unbeknown to my parents I have carried the Mabukane family's legacy to new heights. The nursing profession became my stepping stone to places as far afield as the United Kingdom, United States of America, Asia, and many countries on the African continent. I have travelled to these places with the confidence that I gained from having a solid and loving family background. By ordinary South African standards, we were not rich but were not poor either, which is why this book should inspire young people to travel, see the world, gain confidence and change their mindset. As they say, your attitude determines your altitude.

CHAPTER 2

THE NURSING PROFESSION—MY STEPPING STONE

My professional nurse's training has been my ticket in and out of South Africa to the many countries and stories shared in this book. I trained as a nurse because I was motivated by my cousin, Pathiwe, and because my parents could not afford to send me to university. In those days there were only two options if you could not go to university. You either became a teacher or a nurse. I went into nursing because of the added advantage of getting paid whilst you are on training. This payment came in handy in a family of six children, which was managed by a father who was a primary school teacher and a mother who was a domestic worker. My brother, Ntobeko, was at university, and my sister, Nokuthula was in the same boarding that I had attended. I actually fell in love with the nursing profession, little knowing that it would open so many opportunities and enable me to travel to so many places.

I started my nursing training in July1971 at Frere Hospital in East London. On the first day I was assigned a patient to wash. At 19 years of age, I had never washed an adult before. In those days, there was no orientation and you only survived by working as a team and learning from the senior nurses. The biggest shock that month was learning how to lay out a corpse. I had never seen a dead person and I was scared to touch him. The lead-up to this procedure was more shocking. Mandisa, the senior nurse I worked with, poked and pushed the patient as she told me: "Temsana (her nickname for me), even if this was the scariest person, there is nothing he can do to you now." That is all I learned and I have laid out many dead people since then.

Besides that, I enjoyed my three years of training. For the first time I was free to do as I pleased with my spare time. I did all the things that young people did in those days. As a group that started in the same month, we became friends. We partied a lot and also studied very hard. We could not wait to graduate and be professional nurses or nursing sisters as they were called in those days.

It was whilst in training that I made history in my family. I became the first person to travel by aeroplane. The 30-minute flight from East London to Port Elizabeth to my grandmother's funeral was the first of many trips I would take around the globe. The excitement and wonder in my family made them temporarily forget the sorrow of losing my paternal grandmother. Mostly, people could not believe my courage in risking travel by air.

The truth was that I was on night duty that week and had to request to be off on that particular weekend. I did not have enough time to travel to Hankey by public transport.
The return trip was R17, which is unbelievable compared to the over-R500 that it costs nowadays for the same trip. The reality was that after paying for the ticket I was left with only R18 from my R35 monthly salary, but it was worth it.

We wrote our general nursing diploma examination in June of 1974. We all applied to different institutions in the country for the next certificate, which was a diploma in midwifery. I did not apply to Frere Hospital as I wanted to experience a different environment. I applied to places that I never knew existed, like Sabie in Mpumalanga.

On the day the results came out, I was called to the matron's office. I thought I was going to be congratulated. The matron told me that she had been asked for a reference by one of the hospitals where I had applied. She had looked through my file and found reports which said that I had been "cheeky and stubborn", and she could therefore not recommend me.

I knew exactly who had written that report even without seeing it. In those days; performance evaluation was secretive and subjective. I recalled the incidence that got me the cheeky and stubborn report. It was in the surgical ward. One of the patients, a naughty eight-year-old boy, had lost the inner tube of his tracheostomy. This is a hole that is made in the neck to enable a patient to breath when they have problems breathing normally.

The inserted tube has an inner one that is taken out regularly to be cleaned. Often children feel irritated by these tubes and as they cough, the inner tube may come out and even get lost. This happened on a Friday afternoon as we were preparing to go off duty. The group that took over from us was already in the ward; however the Sister in charge insisted that we all have a lecture on the importance of the procedure, even though the inner tube was found. I did not mean to be rude or to be defiant, but the incident took place on a Friday afternoon. I could already see the cars in front of the nurses' home. They were there to take us for a party at Leaches Bay. With that in mind, I left the ward. That is what earned me the bad report.

The good part of the meeting with the matron was that she offered me a midwifery training post at Frere Hospital, the only one in my group to get it. She felt that I needed some disciplining before letting me loose out into the world. I did not disappoint her. I passed my midwifery diploma examination with honours, which earned me a professional nurses post in the same hospital that I had tried to run away from.
I ended up spending 10 years at Frere Hospital. During this time, like most of my colleagues, I studied for my Bachelor of Arts and Nursing Science Degree, commonly known as BA CUR through correspondence with the University of South Africa. We were all aiming to leave the wards and be tutors on completion. However, tutors' posts were not easily available as they were not people who were changing jobs frequently.

I worked for some time in the clinical teaching department at Frere Hospital after completing my degree in 1982. I worked with many student nurses and it is this interaction that gave me an opportunity to get out of the hospital. This came through one of my former students who I saw in a navy-blue suit and a white shirt. I quickly asked her where she was working and she told me that she was working for the National Department of Health in Community Geriatric Services. She also told me that they were looking for a black professional nurse to start the programme in Duncan Village, one of the oldest townships in East London. I knew nothing about geriatric nursing but I applied on the same day. I was offered the post and this time I was given a full orientation. That was how I ended up driving up and down Duncan Village in a

navy-blue suit, visiting old people and giving them their
monthly medication for chronic diseases.

A second nurse was employed and together we came out with
a plan to do more than just visit the elderly at home. One of
the things that was clear, during the visits, was that the elderly
people were lonely. Some had been left alone as family
members were at work and the children were at school. We
decided to start an initiative where the elderly would come
together once a week and we would check their blood
pressures and also provide them with soup for the day. This
became a highlight in their lives as they were able to socialise
with other old people that they had not seen in a long time.
We would get donations of meat bones from the Cambridge
Butchery and the supermarkets around town donated
vegetables as well as bread.

I loved my job and enjoyed working with the elderly, however
after a year I had to leave with no job in hand and with only
my pride. The whole thing started after my BA CUR
graduation. It was in May 1983 when I was already working in
the Community Geriatric programme. A white colleague, my
supervisor, graduated on the same day with a diploma from
the same university. She was promoted from a senior to a
chief professional nurse after graduation. She motivated for
me to be promoted to a senior professional nurse. The
response she got, which she showed me, was what made me
resign. It was the simple statement that: "There is no senior
position for a black nurse". That was the South Africa of the
eighties.

I stayed at home for two months without a job. I soon learned
that pride does not pay the bills. As I was waiting for my

pension pay-out and a post from the-then Ciskei Government health department, bills had to be paid - especially furniture bought on hire purchase. My husband, Mncedisi, was a high school teacher and could not cope with all the accounts that had been initiated based on two salaries. Although I went to all the shops and explained the situation, I received a telegram informing me that one of the furniture shops, where we had bought a lounge and a bedroom suite, was coming to re--possess the furniture. A friend came to visit us at the time when my husband and I were still trying to come terms with the fact that our neighbours would watch as our beautiful furniture was being repossessed. We told him about our problem. He referred us to one of the lawyers where he worked.

It took the lawyer one phone call and the message that "if you repossess my client's furniture tomorrow, I will see you in court". He then assisted me with claiming my pension, which took a shorter period of time than it would have if I had claimed it personally and we settled the accounts. The incident also taught me of one of the rights that we black people were not aware of. Many people in the township had their furniture re-possessed without knowing that the shops had no legal right to do so.

Shortly after that I was offered a position as a tutor at Mount Coke Hospital. At last, I was a tutor, teaching what I had passed with honours, midwifery. I realised then that I loved teaching and have been in love with it ever since. Mount Coke was far from my home in Mdantsane. I had to take four taxis when I did not have a car. Fortunately, a colleague who stayed in Zwelitsha wanted to swop with me and I ended up in

Cecilia Makiwane Nursing College, which was five minutes away from my house.

Cecilia Makiwane was a big establishment with lots of groups, cliques, gossip and professional jealousy. I ended up in charge of the clinical teaching department again. I made it my business to overhaul it. I converted a storeroom into a library and made sure that the professional nurses working in the clinical department were able to sit together around the table for their meetings and the planning of the procedures that they were going to demonstrate to the students.

One of the challenges that the clinical department had, was of students not finishing the number of procedures, they are supposed to do under supervision, in a year. It was a requirement of the South African Nursing Council (SANC) and it had to be completed before they were allowed to write their examination and move to the next year of their training.

The problem was that nobody was responsible for any group of students. I assigned each group to a clinical nurse who was responsible for making sure that their group completed the required procedures on time. To make sure that there was no resistance to the plan, I assigned the most stubborn one to be in charge of the first group and the others followed suite. The problem was solved.

Whilst at Cecilia Makiwane Hospital, tutors were offered an opportunity to study psychiatric nursing in seven months. There was to be one month of theory, followed by six months of practical training at Komani Psychiatric Hospital. I did not finish the course and only did the one month of theory. Before returning to Komani after the theory month, I received a call that changed my life. The person in charge at the National Department of Health, where I had worked as a geriatric nurse, phoned me to offer me a position as a Chief Professional Nurse. This was a promotion as all the tutors were senior professional nurses. It made me realise that if you take a stand against what you feel is unjust, people will remember that and respect you for it.

CHAPTER 3

AN OPPORTUNITY TO LEARN AND TO SERVE

My appointment - in what was called the Trust Areas - enabled me to find my second love: community-based primary health care. I worked with other supervisors: Sis Nomathemba Faba, Nomusa Fikelepi and Thandi Bebelele. We were supervising seven rural clinics, (Kwelega, Mooiplaas, Soto, Newlands, Needs Camp, Mgwali and Lessyton outside Queenstown), two school health teams and a community psychiatric service.

I loved my job and enjoyed the contact with community members, setting up clinic health committees and health days. I learned an important lesson that community members are able to take care of their own health and our role as health-care workers is to intervene only when their health has broken down.

This was demonstrated when they asked one of the staff nurses to go to the circumcision school at night, something which is taboo in the Xhosa culture. They asked her to give their schizophrenic young man who was in the circumcision school his monthly Modecate Concentrate injection, which is particularly useful in the maintenance treatment of chronic patients who are unreliable at taking their oral medication. The family feared that without the injection, he would relapse, have a mental breakdown and be admitted to a mental hospital. It was better to have a woman, contrary to the culture, go and give him his injection and prevent a mental breakdown

The Health Days became a highlight for each clinic team, with the nurses competing to have the biggest and the best gathering. In addition to the health talks given, there were meals prepared with community members donating the food and cooking. Local shop owners and rich community members, such as Mr. George Qhinga, in Mgwali, donated sheep to be slaughtered and eaten on the Health Days.

The agenda was sent to the community leaders in advance to make sure that those on the programme could prepare. Some community meetings were held on Saturdays. This was usually an outing for me and my husband. For one of the meetings, I sent the agenda to the community leaders as usual. On the agenda items I had written ANC, as an abbreviation for a talk on Ante Natal Care. The agenda ended up with the police and the meeting was cancelled. I was warned by some community members not to come near Newlands Clinic where the meeting was to be held. Only then did it dawn on me that the police interpreted the 'ANC' on the agenda as the African National Congress. That was the South Africa of the late eighties.

In the Trust Areas health services, I trained community health workers and had illiterate women providing health care in areas where nurses were not available. They would give their reports orally and I was intrigued by their indigenous knowledge and management of conditions, especially the delivery of babies. How they made sure that the deliveries were hygienic and the women in labour were kept warm throughout the delivery, impressed me.

All the Trust Area clinics provided a 24-hour service, which meant that nurses stayed in the nurses home next to the clinics. We made their living quarters as comfortable as possible. Their husbands and boyfriends were allowed to visit them and even spend weekends with them. They provided local communities with services when they needed them, and in return the community members were very protective of the nurses, with clinic committees active in the affairs of the establishment.

I was therefore surprised when, as the person in charge of the clinics, I received a message that the Soto Clinic Committee wanted to see me. The meeting was on a Saturday and, as usual, my husband accompanied me. We were planning to drive to Haga Haga after the meeting, which is a seaside holiday resort not far from Soto Clinic.

As we were driving out to Soto, my husband remarked on how far the place was (about 66 km) from East London. This made me appreciate the nurses who stayed there for two weeks before getting a long weekend off. When we arrived, the clinic committee members started the meeting. They were happy with the nurses but were unhappy with one of the staff nurses. According to them, she was having an affair with the white man who came to service the septic tanks and do minor repairs in the clinic. They claimed to have proof of this, as the man was seen leaving the clinic on a particular morning and his car had been parked there for the night. This had been happening for some time now.

I worked in the Trust Areas from 1986 to 1991. During this time, I studied for a Diploma in Nursing Administration with the

University of South Africa. I also registered for an Honours Degree, however I did not complete my studies. I just could not bring myself to study Nursing Ethos again in my honour's degree. It had been part of the basic degree and the diploma I had studied. Whilst in limbo as far as studying was concerned, a friend - Lulu Nkonzo-Mthembu - suggested that I register for a masters degree with the University of Natal which I did. I struggled to travel to Durban every month for the meetings with Professor Uys, my supervisor, as I did not have any financial support.

The same friend, who was studying for her doctorate at the time, told me that she had a secured a British Council scholarship and she was going to the United Kingdom for a six-week study period. She advised me to apply for the same programme, which I did. All went well with my application and the British Council team set a date to come to East London for the interview. I phoned my friend to help me prepare for the interview. She told me, in no uncertain terms, that I needed to change my application from six weeks to a year for a masters programme. I was shocked and scared. What if the request was turned down?

The interview went well and I could see that the team was impressed with my responses and my knowledge of primary health care and community work. It is only when they asked me if I had any questions that I dropped the bombshell. I told them that I actually wanted to study for a masters degree. They were taken aback by this change of direction and said so. They wanted the name of the university where I wanted to study, of course I had no idea as I had not prepared for the question. They asked me to write another motivation letter and state where I wanted to study and the reasons for choosing that particular university.

Although I had started the interview feeling confident, I was left feeling very unsure of myself and not knowing whether I would get the bursary or not. I applied to the University of Liverpool for my masters degree in community health and, as they say, the rest is history. I was to start at Liverpool University on the 6th of January 1992.

The last quarter of 1991 went off as if I was in a dream. Big decisions had to be made about my 11-year-old daughter Pinky, my 71-year-old father Lizo, and my sickly mother, Nobandla, who had just had a stroke. There were also my siblings: my elder brother Mthuthuzeli and my sisters Thula, Connie and Zoliswa. There was also my government-subsidised house in Gompo Township, in East London, and my job in the Trust Areas. All these thoughts gave me sleepless nights.

Much as I was excited, I was also scared. I got through all this with the support of my family, who were all excited for me. I had again made history in my family and I would be the first one to go overseas. Again, the apartheid government did not disappoint. The response to my application for the study leave, which was well motivated by my supervisor, Rina Blundell, was one sentence, namely "dit is nie goed gekeur," meaning that it was not approved. This meant that I had to make a decision about my professional career. Do I resign a highly sought-after Chief Professional Nurse's position and go and study? I remember a friend and colleague, Sis Nomathemba Faba, who found me deep in thought in my office. I told her about my dilemma. She brought me a card

30

and the words in the card were simple but powerful. It simply said: "Whatever decision you make, I will support you." Those words made me strong in my resolve to resign from my job, sell my house, pack my bags and go to school at the age of 39.

On the 16th of December 1991, friends and relatives threw me a big party and had a sheep slaughtered. Everybody was excited. My sisters Thula and Connie came from Port Elizabeth for the party. Zoliswa brought me the biggest suitcase I had ever seen as a present. She also promised to take good care of Pinky in my absence and I did not doubt this as I knew how much she loved her. Pinky, my daughter, was the only person who was not happy with the whole things. She felt, and later told me, that I had abandoned her. I felt guilty but reckoned that opportunities like these were few and came once in a person's life. I explained to her that the whole trip was aimed at us having a better life later on. How that would happen, I had no idea, but knew that whatever I said made no sense to an eleven-year-old.

Getting the scholarship to study in Liverpool was a result of friends who mean well and supported me with progressing along my career path. We all need such friends. Lulu was, and still is, that friend who motives me.

CHAPTER 4

FIRST JOURNEY OUT OF SOUTH AFRICA

My trip to the United Kingdom was my first trip outside the borders of South Africa. I left home on one of the hottest days on the 3rd of January 1992 to study at the Liverpool University's School of Tropical Medicine, sponsored by the British Council.

When I arrived at Heathrow Airport I had imagined that it was going to be cold but never thought it could be that cold. As I walked out of the airport it felt like icy arms were embracing me. It was such a shock that I retreated back into the airport building. I had a beautiful long coat that I had bought from one of the second-hand shops in East London for the trip. At the time, it had felt ridiculous buying a coat in the middle of December. However, at that moment it felt like I had only a shirt on.

I stayed a few minutes in the airport building, thinking that there was no need to rush out as there was no one waiting for me on the outside. This was a complete contrast to when I left home where friends and family had hired a 14-seater taxi - for those who did not have cars - to see me off at the airport. I had clear instructions that I had printed and put in my handbag which told me exactly where to go from the airport.

I had struggled to haul my big suitcase from the conveyer belt and now had to drag it, and other pieces of luggage, to the underground train to travel to the city. I learned my first lesson about travelling light as I walked from the train station to the British Council offices in London. At the offices, I was handed my settling allowance and the train fare for my one-way ticket to Liverpool.

The two young men who took me to the station did not once assist me with my luggage. The speed at which they left me at the station made me feel as if they could not get away fast enough from this woman who seem to have brought the whole of Africa to England in her suitcase. I struggled along with my big suitcase, reading notices on the wall and overhead. I found the booth where I bought the ticket and waited at the platform for the train, just glad that nobody knew me.

The trip to Liverpool felt like the whole day, instead of only three hours, as I sat in one place to keep warm. I later learned that there were hot beverages served but was too cold and glued to my seat to notice anything. Travelling through mostly beautiful green fields with dams and ponds, we finally arrived at Liverpool Station. According to my instructions I was to take a taxi to an address in Liverpool 48. I later learned that the area was home to the Liverpool Football Club team members who won the World Football Cup in that year. The taxi driver, who I could not understand at first because of his accent which I later learned was a "Scouse's, or Liverpudlian" accent, was kind enough to help me with my luggage.

The road to my first home in Liverpool was a blur of tall buildings that left me wondering how I would survive in such a cold place. The taxi driver dropped me at a building that looked like a hostel. My anticipation of a warm room and cup of hot coffee was shattered by the notice on the door of the office. It stated that the place was closed and would only open at 4pm, two hours from the time of my arrival. I stood alone on the veranda, shaking from head to toe because of the cold wind that came from the lake at the bottom of the building. As I could not stand the cold anymore, I did a typical African thing. I opened my big suitcase I pulled out a scarf and wrapped it around my head and face, leaving only my eyes not covered. I asked myself a question that I have asked myself many times in different countries: "What the hell am I doing here?"

Feeling a bit warmer, I started noticing my surrounding and noticed warmly dressed young girls going in and out of the building and then out of the gate. My typical South African apartheid mentality did not give me enough courage to ask for help from these young white girls. It is only when I saw a black girl that I mustered the courage and asked when the office would open, even though I knew. I suppose I was embarrassed to ask for help outright.

I automatically addressed her in Xhosa and her puzzled look made me realise that she might be black but not necessarily Xhosa speaking. I asked the question again in English. She must have seen the desperation in my face and my shaking body so she promised to take me to her room on her return from the shops. True to her word, the girl, whose name I later learned was Nancy and she was from Kenya, came back and took me to her warm room. She offered me a most appreciated cup of coffee.

The office finally opened at 4pm and I was given the key to my room, where I would stay until the following day, Monday, when I would move to the university residents where I stayed until June. Nancy took me to the shops to buy food and - most importantly coffee, sugar and milk - which I drank almost throughout the night as I was too cold to fall asleep immediately. This was even though the room had central heating and I was tired. All I could think about was my daughter, Pinky. I missed her. I missed my parents, my sisters and all my friends.

I had applied for university residence close to the School of Tropical Medicine where I would be studying. Applying from home in South Africa, the place made sense to me as I had no one to ask. Little did I know that it was one of the most expensive places. Most of my classmates were staying in residences that were not far from the school but cheaper. I shared the university apartment with five other students, all younger than me. It was a two multi-storied building with one boy on the ground floor, myself and two other girls having rooms on the first floor and two boys on the upper floor. We shared the living room and the kitchen. The place was cleaned twice a week by an elderly white lady, something my mother - who had been a domestic worker all her life - could not believe.

The first day at school was an eye-opener. To start with, this was the first time I was a full-time university student. I was the only student from South Africa. There were many students from Africa and even the white students in the class had worked in Africa. We had been asked to prepare a presentation on the health-care services in our respective countries. The discussions were like a scene from the English comedy: "Mind Your Language". It was the first time I had heard so many different accents and I was fascinated.

I had worked hard on my presentation at home, but at the time it was difficult to clearly describe health services in the country as they were about to change and take a different direction. In 1992, black people were a government in waiting. I had been an active member of the National Progressive Primary Health Care Network (NPPHCN) which focused on changing the health-care system from the curative and hospi-centric health care system to a primary health care system as envisaged by the incoming ANC government.

However, I had to describe the current system, which was well resourced where the shortage of drugs was an unknown phenomenon. I had worked in the Eastern Cape where we had more than 13 health-care providers including the National Department of Health, the Cape Provincial Administration, the Transkei, and Ciskei Homelands Health Departments and a number of municipal health services.

The presentations by the student from other African countries were like horror stories - of services with no drugs, no gloves and no sterile needles and no medication. Little did I know that one day we would also be without gloves in our facilities. I also learned of terms that I had never heard before, like the International Monetary Fund (IMF), the World Bank, Structural Adjustments and Acquired Immunodeficiency Syndrome (AIDS). One student actually worked in an AIDS project in Uganda. In 1991 and before, little was known and discussed about AIDS in South Africa. We were just not talking about it.

We were busy talking about our freedom, a topic that generated a lot of interest from my classmates. I would hold the floor during our ritual pub visits on Friday afternoons after class. We had our own Class of 1992 pub, which was chosen by an Irish fellow student. One of the questions asked by my fellow students, about South African politics, was: "Why was Mandela negotiating with the Whites?" I must confess, at the time, I was unable to answer the question.

I quickly made friends and my closest friends were the three students from Zimbabwe, perhaps because of their proximity to home. I had no idea about any other country. The Zimbabweans use to call me Mandela's Child (Mntana Ka Mandela) and I called them Mugabe's Children (abantwana bakaMugabe). I felt closer to Dorothy Dhliwayo, who spoke Ndebele, which is similar to the Zulu language. Robert Mugabe was still very popular then, although it was his 12th year in power. In particular, the one student - Ruth Labode, who had been a freedom fighter and had trained as a doctor in Bulgaria - was very militant and full of praise for 'Bob' as she called Mugabe. The other two nurses were not so enthusiastic. They were already talking about the shortages of specific goods in Zimbabwe. They even packed boxes of matches in the parcels that they sent home. They all criticised what, I now know, to be our negotiated settlement in South Africa. I later wished I could meet them after we were free and Zimbabwe was plunged into the disaster that it is now in.

The masters programme in Liverpool was structured into five modules and included three months of research in a developing country that you were not familiar with. This was what had attracted me to the Liverpool programme in the first place. I liked the idea of travelling.

I struggled with the first module as my research background was not that strong. The other modules were based on actual community health work which I had been doing in the rural health services I had worked in before leaving home. In working on my assignments, I drew from my experiences of the Kwelega, Mooiplaas, Soto, Newlands, Mgwali and Lessyton clinics. Those experiences helped me to theorise what I had been doing without being able to put a name to it. The modules included planning, implementation, monitoring and evaluation of health services.

One of the advantages of the community health programme at the University of Liverpool is the fact that the lecturers are involved in projects in different developing countries. This meant that their experiences were practical and relevant. This is so different from the local nursing colleges where most lecturers are not aware of what is happening in the service delivery areas.

The most interesting part of the programme was conducting research in a developing country that I was not familiar with. Four countries had sent topics and invited the students to conduct the research in their countries. These countries were Ghana, Fiji, Tanzania and Nepal. I was drawn to one of the topics on community health workers in Fiji and also chose the country because the name fascinated me. However, one of the lecturers advised me that there was not much I would learn about Fiji as it was similar to South Africa in terms of development. He advised me to choose an African country and, as I was drawn to a topic on AIDS, he suggested Ghana.

My trips to Liverpool and Ghana confirmed what a friend once said: "You must travel the world whilst you can still sleep in your jeans". This is something I always tell young people when I am motivating them to study overseas.

CHAPTER 5

MY FIRST VISIT TO ANOTHER COUNTRY IN AFRICA

My research topic - which was "Exploring Entry Avenues for HIV/AIDS education amongst out of School Youths in Ghana" - was requested by the Ghanaian government. During the beginning of literature review in Liverpool, I discovered that studies on HIV and AIDS had been conducted by Professor Coovadia and other South Africans way back in the 1980s. The problem was that, at the time, there was limited access to information in South Africa. Also, technology was not as advanced as it is today. The research proposals were presented to the whole class and a panel of lecturers. Good feedback was given which made me feel confident about my topic and research methods as the days went by.

As we prepared for our travels and research in the different countries, we were assigned to different lecturers who would travel with us to the countries as our supervisors. The lecturers were chosen according to their knowledge of the countries. The Ghana group was assigned to Dave, an easy-going Irish man. The school made our travel arrangements.

Six of us were to travel to Ghana, three French students, one Spanish girl, one Bangladeshi doctor and myself, being the only African.

I was shocked when I was denied a visa to Ghana. I did not know that African countries had forbade South Africans from travelling to their countries as part of their support in the fight against Apartheid. Dave assured me that he would travel with the other five students and arrange my visa from Ghana. As he put it: "I will tell them that you are a black South African."

The delay in my visa meant that all my classmates travelled to Ghana, Fiji, Tanzania and Nepal and I was left with one classmate from Afghanistan who was unable to get a visa from any of the countries. The school made travel arrangements that were cost effective which made the trip longer but also meant travelling through other countries. In my case, I travelled from Manchester to Schiphol Airport in the Netherlands, then to Kano in Northern Nigeria and finally to Kotoka Airport in Accra in Ghana. From admiring the beauty of Schiphol Airport, I got my first African culture shock at Kano Airport. For the first time I saw passengers literally running towards the aircraft. The was no order with boarding according to seat numbers - just first come first served. Whilst watching all this through the aeroplane window, I lost my camera which was on the seat next to me. There was nobody to ask and therefore the end of taking photos until I could buy another one.

My classmates and Dave were at the airport to meet me and waved as I walked into the terminal building, which made me feel at home. At immigration the first West African experience happened. I was asked for my yellow immunisation booklet, with all the immunisations that I had received in the Liverpool Travel clinic. I could clearly see it in the suitcase that I checked in with my luggage. As I mumbled an explanation to the immigration officer, he simply put my passport aside without stamping it.

As I hopelessly stood there, I noticed that as some passengers handed him their passports, he would take out money notes from the passports and stamp them. That is when all the stories I had heard about West Africa came to my mind. I distinctly remember the one about "page 20 is missing from your passport". I realised that my page 20 was my yellow book. I behaved like a typical South African township girl. I took my passport, put in two ten-pound notes and confidently announced: "Sir, I have found my yellow book". The officer did not even look up, he simply stamped my passport and I was through immigration.

Just like the cold I felt on landing at Heathrow airport had enveloped me with icy hands, the heat at Kotoka Airport hit me like a brick. The friendly black faces around me and the welcome hugs from my classmates immediately made me feel at home. This is a feeling I still have whenever I land in any country on the African continent - except perhaps in Nigeria. Having said that, my first visit to an African country was another culture shock.

England was not a culture shock for me - the food, the cars and the highways were familiar. Even the nightclubs we frequented in Liverpool 28 were like township parties with lots of drinks and familiar music. Ghana was different. The sight of men in beautiful colourful cloths, thrown over their shoulders with strong black arms out, fascinated me. The music was wonderful highlife music but the food was my lowest point. I could not get used to the Kenke, Yam and Fufu and had to stick to Jolof rice, meat and vegetables. I immediately developed diarrhoea in the hotel where we were staying in Accra. That is when I learned of the healing power of paw paw for an upset stomach. The waiter at the hotel suggested it when he learned of my plight and I have used it ever since then.

The following day, being a Sunday, we went out to Labadi Beach. We had lots of fun which for me was only spoiled when they started playing a Lucky Dube's song, "Going back to my roots". I cried when I realised that I had been away from home for nearly six months.

We stayed till late at the beach resort and realised that we were all out of money for the taxi to get back to the hotel. Dave, the resourceful Irish man, negotiated with a truck driver who bundled all of us on the back of his trunk, which did not matter as we were all going back to the same hotel.

On Monday the work started. Dave took me to the Ministry of Health and the Director of the HIV and Aids programme in the country. It was fascinating to see a black female doctor in such a high position as that. Remember that, in 1992, we black South Africans were nowhere near those seats of power yet. She suggested that I conduct my research in the eastern region of the country, whose capital is Koforidua. However, she suggested that I first visit the Volta Region, which was not only the hardest hit by AIDS but was also over researched.

I travelled to the Volta Region the following day and spent the night with another female doctor who was the district manager. She took me to the nearest hospital, where I saw - for the first time - patients with AIDS and patients dying from AIDS. I, as a professional nurse from South Africa, saw an AIDS patient for the first time in 1992, not knowing that - 10 years later - I would see so many of my friend, relatives and even family members die from AIDS.

Back in Accra, Dave decided to review my research plan at the local drinking spot and made sure that the barman would take care of me in any future visits. He accompanied me to the Eastern Region Health Department and introduced me to my local supervisor, Dr Dela Dovlo, the regional director. Dela was a very warm and supportive supervisor who helped me to understand the nuances of a foreign culture as I worked through my research plan and questionnaires. He introduced me to his wife who helped with my food problem, cooking familiar dishes that I really enjoyed. I later met Dela Dovlo in Bellagio, Italy in 1999, when we attended a Ford Foundation-sponsored Human Resources Management conference.

Dr Dovlo invited me to attend a district health management committee meeting. The meeting was an eye-opener for me as I had no point of reference. We did not have such things in South Africa before 1994. I also appreciated how non-governmental organisations (NGOs) and community members participated in the meetings and made meaningful contributions to the discussions. This was not the case at home where NGOs still operated secretly in 1992.

The following day, which was a Saturday, we travelled to Dela's rural home on the Gulf of Guinea. Seeing people cramped in small rowing boats and going about their business made me realise how resilient people are in Africa.

I conducted my research in the Eastern Region where the biggest town was Koforidua. I stayed in a village called Obomeng which is in Nkwankaw, the capital town of the Kwahu West Municipality. An Irish lady who worked for an NGO in the area invited me to Obomeng and organised a place for me to stay. I stayed in one of the rich men's houses. The owner was in Accra and there was a houseboy, an old man actually who looked after the house. He took very good care of me and made sure that I had bath water in buckets every morning. He could not understand why I did not want any of the local foods. I had decided that I was not going to risk diarrhoea again, especially in a house with no running water. I survived on local chicken, rice and eggs in the morning.

I had to have my breakfast as I was taking anti-malaria tablets every morning. The one time I took them on an empty stomach, I regretted it. I had to travel to Koforidua to meet with my supervisor, Dave. Whilst sitting in a 20-seater bus, called a "Troto", waiting for it to fill up to even more than the twenty people already in it.

I looked through the window. The sight of the flies on the meat and fish displayed suddenly nauseated me. I could feel that I was going to vomit and fortunately I was sitting next to the window, but my worry was that I always wet myself whenever I vomit. When the next wave of nausea came, all I could do was to lean through the window and vomit and feel the urine coming out at the same time. What made things worse was that people in the Troto were concerned and many friendly faces came to offer help. The problem was that they we speaking Twi, the local language, and I could not understand a word. I just kept on shaking my head and mumbling that I did not understand. On the way, I thought about the reason why I had exposed myself to all this and at that moment no tangible response came to mind.

Dave travelled with me back to Obomeng to introduce me to the local chief as part of community entry. I could not believe my ears when drums were beaten to call the elders to the palace for my introduction. We were well received. The chief was an Oxford University graduate. It was 1992, yet he asked me to be his third wife - a request which I turned down!

My research went well despite all the trouble of having to translate the questionnaire from English to Twi with the assistance of a local teacher. I presented my questionnaire to Dr Dovlo before administering it. He removed one question, which was: "Have you ever had sex whilst under the influence of alcohol". He felt that the question was not relevant to the Christian community I was working with. This is one question that you cannot omit in any HIV/AIDS-related study that you are conducting on behaviour and practices in South Africa. The research in Ghana was examining knowledge, behaviour and practices around HIV/ AIDS amongst out of school youth to develop avenues for education.
I could afford to employ two translators: a man and a woman. The man worked with the young men who were apprenticed to mechanics and carpenters while the woman worked with the

girls who were apprenticed to the Madams for sewing. What was frustrating was seeing the groups laughing during the focus group discussions and not knowing what they were laughing about. Fortunately, the male translator, a teacher and the lady, a graduate, would debrief me every day.

I did not mention that I was very rich when I was in Ghana. The Liverpool School of Tropical Medicine gave us all £750 for the three months that we were going to be in the field. The Ghanaian Cedi was 269 Cedes to the British Pound Sterling, and even more on the black market. I would change the pounds at the street bureau de change and come back with a bag full of well-used and sometimes dirty notes. I used this money to pay my translators, maintain myself and managed to even send some to my father at home in addition to the monthly allowance I sent to my sister for Pinky's upkeep.

Two and half months in an African community is a long time and you can't avoid becoming part of it. I attended funerals and sat at taverns having long discussions in trying to understand the people. They, on the other hand, wanted to know more about South Africa. I was invited to speak at the local high school. The children were fascinated and impressed with South Africa. One thing that they could not understand was how so many millions of black people were oppressed by a few white people. This I tried to explain to the best of my ability.

Funerals were not held every weekend in Obomeng. Unlike in South Africa, they were held every two weeks. Those who died during the two weeks were all buried over one weekend. This was the weekend when all liquor outlets, shebeens and taverns were stocked to the fullest because people, especially men, would be coming from Accra.

I learned that a man's wealth was measured by the quality of the cloth he wore, and those Accra men were well dressed. I was also lent an outfit to attend a funeral of somebody I did not know. What fascinated me was how people were dancing and celebrating during the funerals, even taking their portable record players - with music blaring - to the graveyard. I was told that the dead person's life was being celebrated. This was unlike what we do at home, where we cry during the burial service and have sessions afterwards where we drink and have "after tears".

One thing that still reminds me of Obomeng is a small spaza shop that was called Mandela. It touched me and made me feel sad when foreigners are treated badly at home as they love us and treat us well in their countries. I also remember the day I dropped my purse - that was full of Ghanaian Cedis - in a taxi. Somebody handed it over to the driver who made a U-turn to give me back my purse. This would be an exceptionally rare occasion in a South African taxi.

The time quickly went by and we had to assemble from all corners of Ghana at the Ministry of Health in Accra to present our research finding to the highest health officials. We all got good feedback and they accepted our recommendations on how to address the issues that we had researched.

The journey back to England was pleasant until we arrived at Manchester Airport. I was pulled out of the queue and my luggage was thoroughly searched. Being a South African, I questioned why I was singled out from the rest of my classmates. I was told that I looked like a Nigerian and all Nigerians were searched for drugs. We had two Nigerian women in my class and I thought I did not look like them. Only when I looked at myself in the mirror did I realise that I had actually gone darker than usual from the sun in Ghana and I had done long braids from the many good salons I had come across in Accra before travelling back to Liverpool.

Back in England we had two weeks to do the write-up, corrections and submission of our dissertation. These were sleepless nights but one of the advantages was the support I got from my local supervisor who was not the same person as the one who went into the field with you. She looked at my research with fresh eyes and gave good feedback. Dave managed to get the Ghana group together for a celebratory party after the submission of our dissertation.

After the research submission, and during the public holidays, I visited a number of places including Wales, London, Manchester and Stratford upon Avon where the Shakespeare Museum is situated. In Liverpool I visited a number of historical sites. I visited the Beatles Museum and the John Lennon Museum which houses the white piano and his guitar. I was also invited by a classmate to her home in Edinburgh in Scotland.

The last two and half months were left for the last module on influencing policy, defending the dissertation and the final examination. One of the people who was on the panel, when I was defending my dissertation, was a South African. From his questions it was clear that we still had a long way in educating the South African community about HIV/AIDS.

The final exam was based on all the work we had done during the year. However, I was still a nervous wreck on the day. I kept on thinking: "What if I failed? What If I had wasted a whole year?" Fortunately, I passed.

I graduated on the 14th of December 1992 and was on a flight home the following day. I arrived at home on a public holiday, the 16th of December, back to sunny South Africa. Another welcome party was held by my sisters and friends, the same people who had thrown me a farewell party. I had to tell all what I had seen and they were more interested in the stories about Ghana. I told them about how I stayed in a beautiful double storey house with no running water. I knew that there were areas in South Africa, like my own village of Krwakrwa in Alice in 1992, where we did not have running water in the house and depended on a communal tap. Little did I know that even those areas which had running water in the townships would be without water for days because of our government that everybody was excited about in 1994.

The Ghana trip made me realise that we have to leave our comfort zones, experience other people's realities to fully understand them and better interact with them.

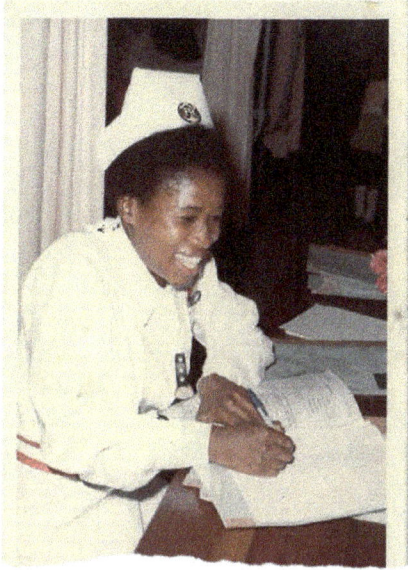

Student Nurse at Frere Hospital

South Africa

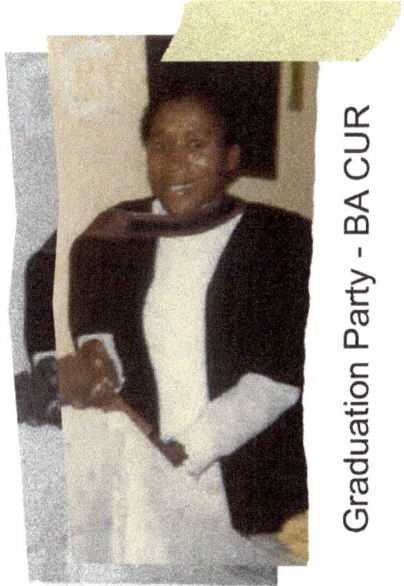

Graduation Party - BA CUR

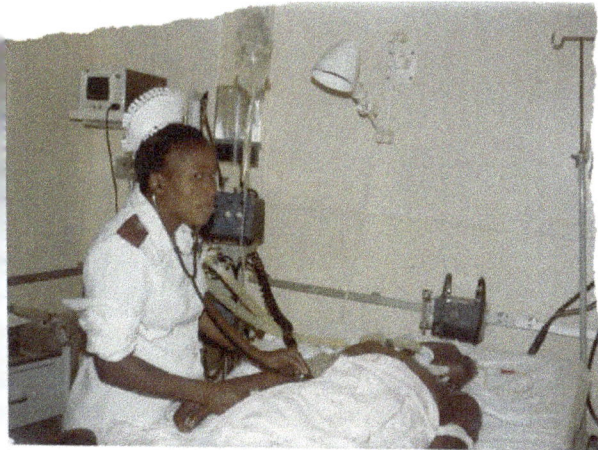

**Professional Nurse
in the Hospital**

Intensive Care Unit
at Frere Hospital

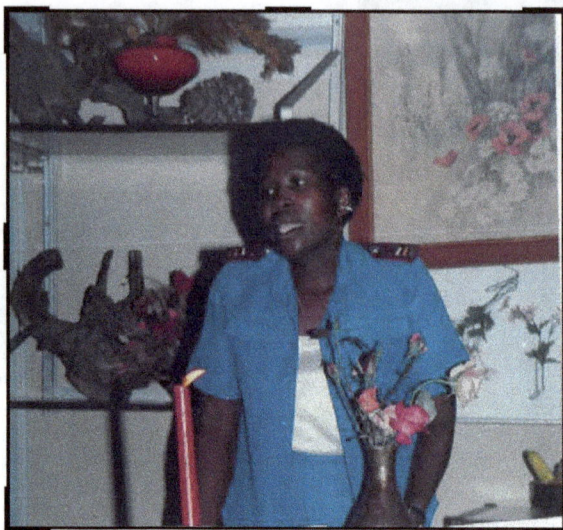

Chief Professional Nurse in the Trust Areas
in the Eastern Cape Province

Border Institute of Primary Health with Staff

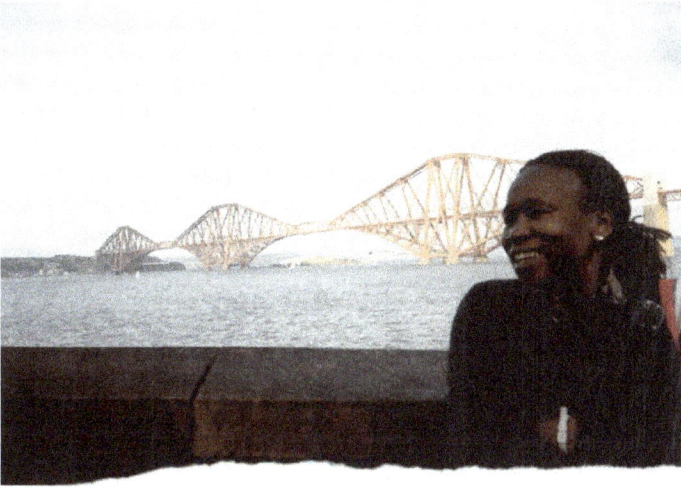

Europe

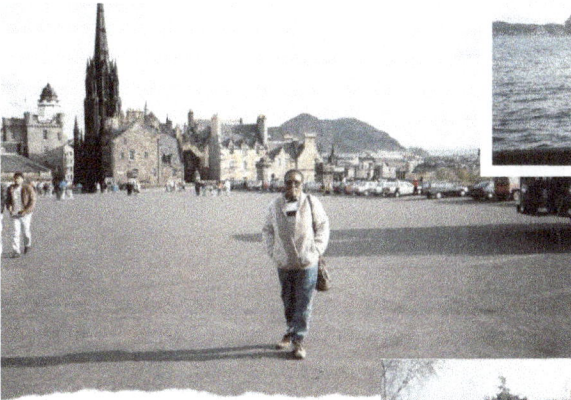

Edinburgh
in Scotland

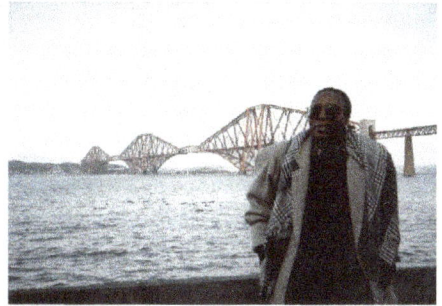

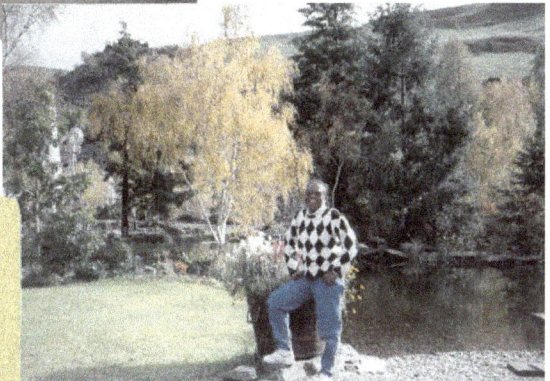

Maghechenttle in Wales

Europe

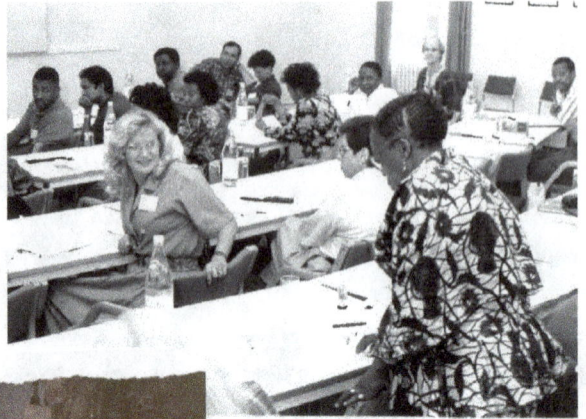

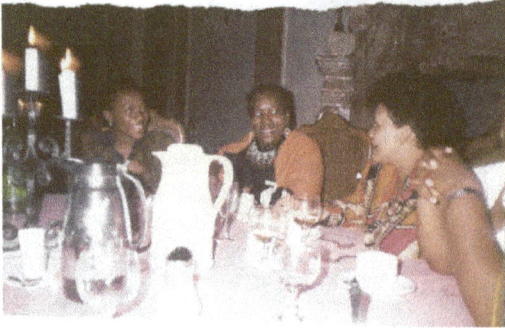

Salzburg Seminar – Austria

Ghana

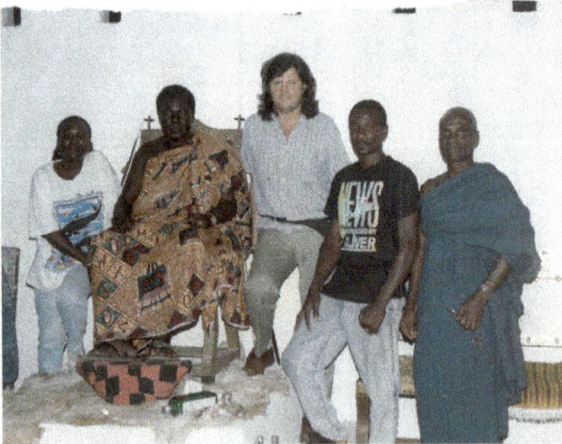

Introduction to the local Chief in Obomeng
with my Field Supervisor

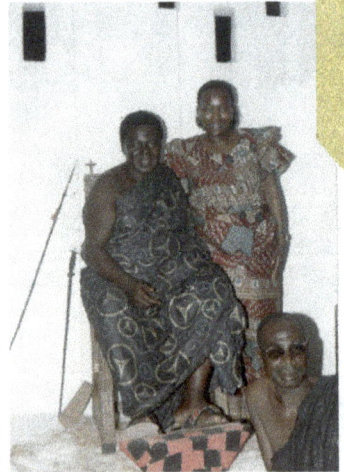

Visit to the Chief of Obomeng

Gulf of Guinea in Ghana

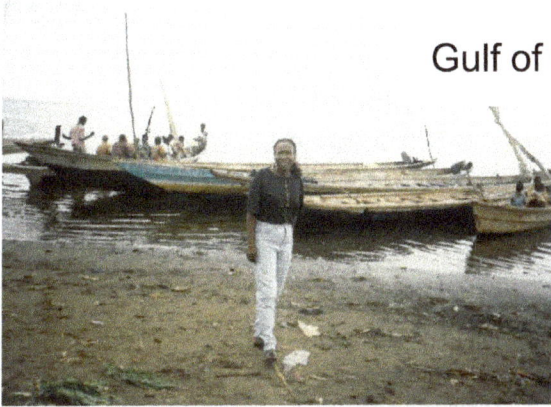

Obomeng Village in Ghana

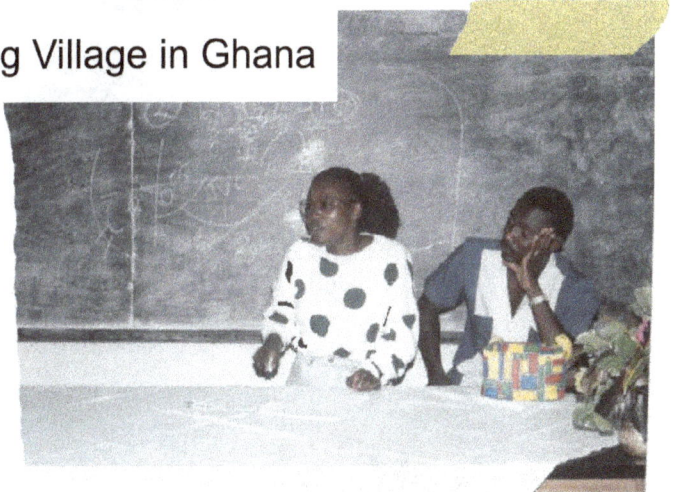

South Africa

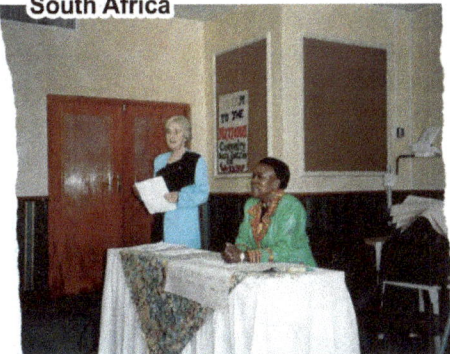

National Community Based Education Workshop in East London in the Eastern Cape Province with former MEC in Health, Dr. Trudy Thomas

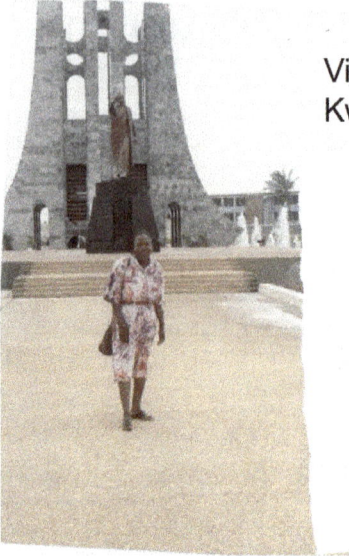

Visit the Statue of
Kwame Nkrumah in Ghana

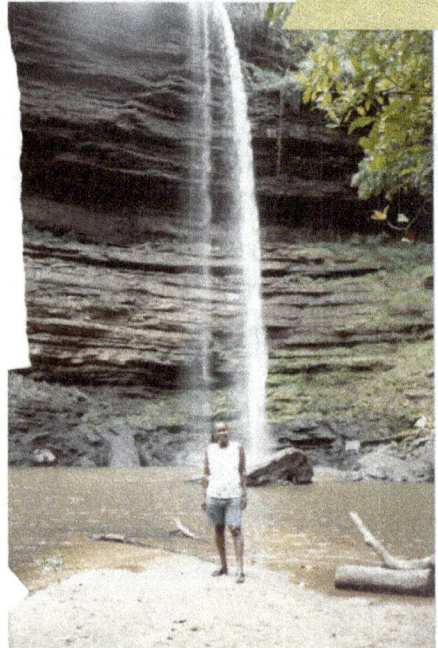

Water Falls in the Eastern Region of Ghana

Mexico City

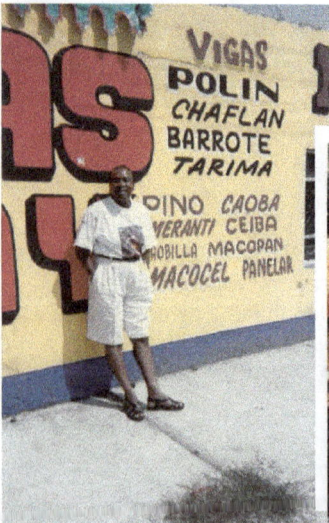

VIGAS
POLIN
CHAFLAN
BARROTE
TARIMA

PINO CAOBA
VERANTI CEIBA
ROBILLA MACOPAN
MACOCEL PANELAR

North & South America

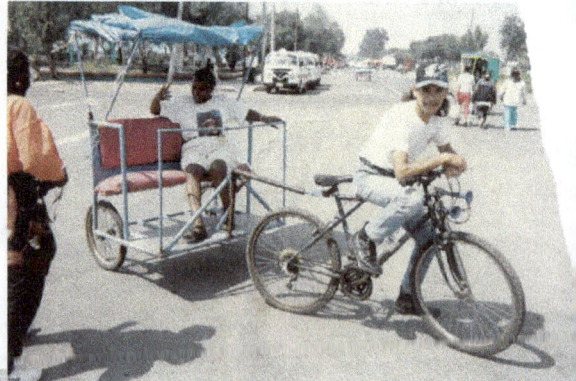

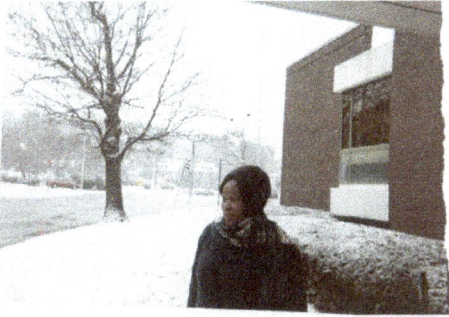

Boston

Miami

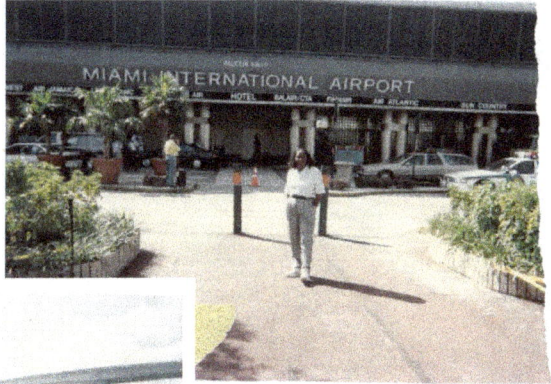

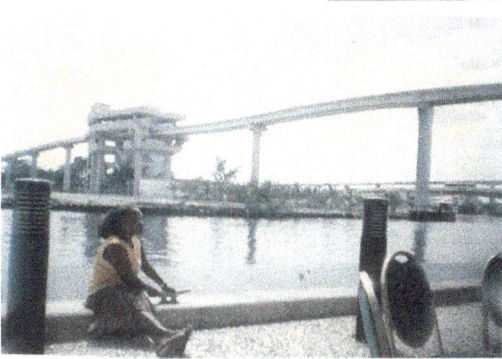

North & South America

Chicago with a friend

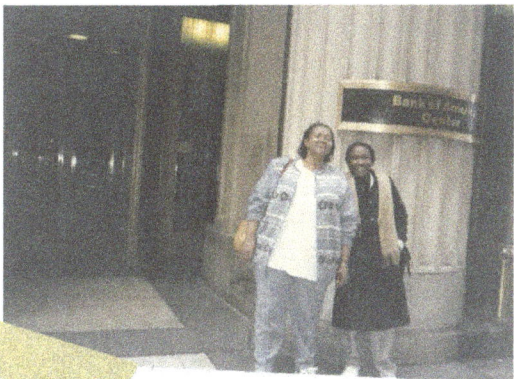

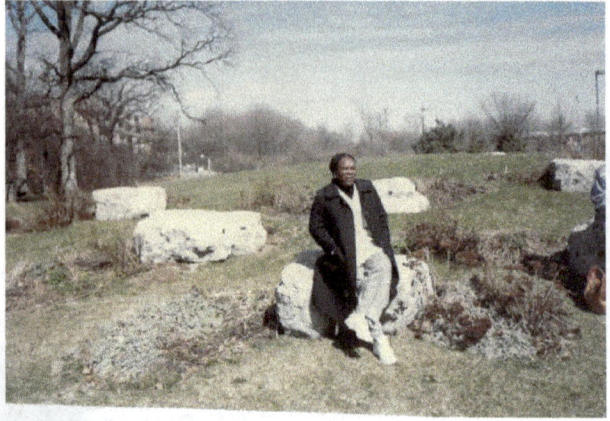

Disneyland Orlando in Florida

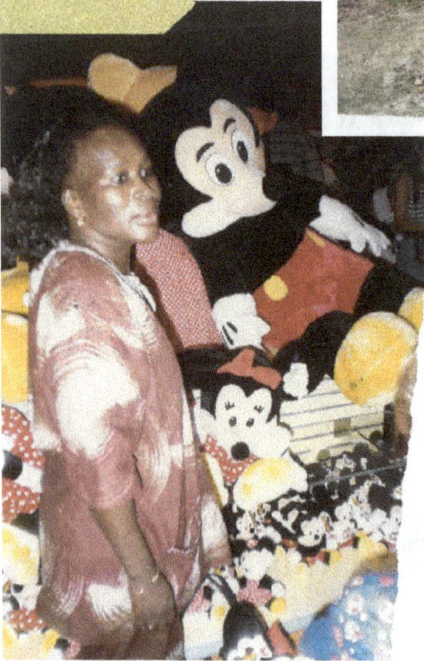

West Virginia

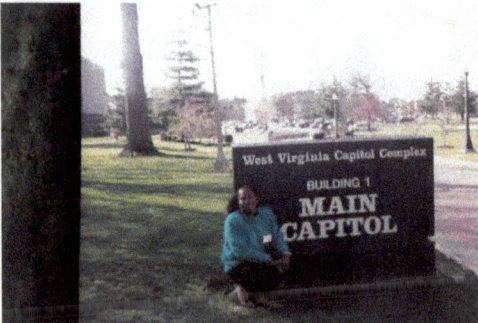

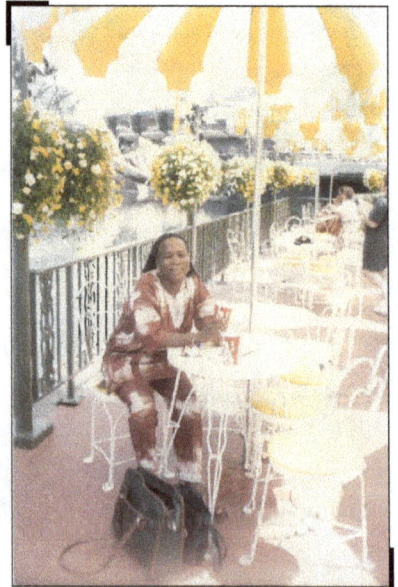

CHAPTER 6

STARTING A COMMUNITY-BASED ORGANIZATION

After the excitement, reality set in. I had a masters degree but no job. I had been able to enjoy the December festivities because of the few pounds I had saved. It was now January 1993 and I had a I had a 12-year-old daughter who was going to start high school. This is where I appreciate my nursing profession. I could take my nursing certificates and the South African Nursing Council (SANC) registration receipt to any health institution and get a job.

I went to St Dominic's Hospital in East London. They were looking for nurses to work on night duty and I was willing to do that as long as I could get paid at the end of the month, as they say beggars can't be choosers. The Matron at St Dominic's was sceptical about people with higher degrees - in her own words: "They used private hospitals as a waiting room, whilst looking for greener pastures." Much as I assured her that I would stay, by the end of the month I was gone. I was recruited by the late Dr Managaliso Maqina to work with Dr Trudy Thomas to start the Border Institute of Primary Health (BIPH).

We started BIPH from scratch. Even the desk and chairs that we used were donated from one of the municipal clinics that was closing. The project was funded by the Kellogg's Foundation as part of an initiative to introduce health care and associated personnel to community-based education (CBE). It was part of 27 other initiatives that they funded. There were seven in South Africa, seven in the United States of America and 13 in South America. The initiative is called Community Partnership in Health Personnel Education (CP-HPE) and is a partnership between health services, training institutions and communities. It was implemented through taking students out of the classroom into the community where they would see a healthy person before they saw sick people.

The BIPH initiative was formed by the Eastern Cape Department of Health (the area called Central Region then), Frere Nursing College, Fort Hare Nursing Science Department and Fort Cox Agricultural College with the community of Newlands. In addition to the student nurses' programme, other programmes included training of community health workers, training nursing assistants at Frere Hospital offering bursaries for health-related studies. CBE is aimed at removing the students from the Ivory Towers to be in the community, albeit for a short time, to see first-hand where their patients came from and where they went back to on discharge.

The concept was easier said than done. Most resistance came from the intellectuals in the training institutions. During combined project meetings and workshops, they were the ones who laboured and argued about decisions to be made. They saw a problem which the community representative did not see. The community members called them the "amantelentele" (Intellectuals).

With students going to the communities, the same communities where they came from, the intellectuals felt that they "would be bitten by snakes". The community members questioned why they were still alive if there were so many snakes in their community. Frere Nursing College students were the first to go to Newlands and thoroughly enjoyed it. They were paired with the local community health workers who taught them so much about the community and how to behave when you are visiting somebody in their homes, which was different from how you treated your patients in hospital.

I enjoyed and learned a lot from the six years that I spent at BIPH. My joy came when students told me how, in their first year, they learned that you have to think twice before discharging an amputee to the village as the toilet was far away. Nurses learned to respect community members as they were visitors in their homes. Communities could see familiar faces in the nurses when they came to Frere Hospital.

In their second year, they learned how the communities dealt with pregnancy and home deliveries at night when there were no ambulances to carry them to the hospital on time. They enjoyed the third year the most when they engaged with traditional healers to understand how they treated their patients with mental health problems as compared to how they were treated in hospital.

In their fourth year they worked at the local clinic. I am proud that the initiative is still alive at Lilitha Nursing College and at the Faculty of Nursing at the University of Fort Hare as well as at many other training institutions throughout the country.

In addition to the student's initiative, other programmes included the training of community health workers. I worked with my former head prefect from Healdtown, Hazel Mangcu, who was the trainer of the community health workers. The project also facilitated the training of nursing assistants at Frere Hospital by paying them a stipend. We trained some of the community health workers to be nursing assistants. It was with a sense of pride that I was invited to a graduation of one of them who had started as a newly wed rural wife ("Makoti"), with a baby on her back, and was now a professional nurse with a four-year diploma. We also assisted others with gaining entrance to professional nurses training at Frere Hospital. To this day, I am greeted by nurses, some of whom I don't even remember, who thank me profusely for the opportunity I gave them to be graduates and professionals.

The Kellogg Foundation, through BIPH, provided bursaries for health-related studies to the Newlands High School. However, the bursary programme hit a snag when we realised that the students did not have science as a subject at the time. Mathematics and science are required subjects for those who wanted to study medicine. We channelled most of the students to the social work programme at the nearby Rhodes University, which had started a branch in East London. Some went to agricultural studies and animal husbandry at Fort Cox College. The students from Fort Cox College assisted the community to establish food gardens. The project educated the community about building toilets and using the public cemeteries instead of burying loved ones in their gardens.

The most important lesson I learned actually started my love for monitoring and evaluation. We were working hard and had good results, however there was no numerical measure of what we called successes. And when the Kellogg Foundation came for an evaluation visit this came sharply to the fore.

When we said that the community had built toilets, they wanted to know the number. How were we to know this when we had not counted them in the beginning? The question on numbers persisted and we had no answers. Although we could mention that there were less diarrhoeal-related deaths as we had taught the communities about the sugar and salt solution to prevent dehydration we still did not have numbers. I knew that we had to start monitoring and documenting whatever we were doing and comparing it with when we had started. That was the start of my lifelong relationship with monitoring, evaluation and health information systems.

Every job has its ups and downs. Mine came when I was phoned by the matron at Frere Hospital. What she said chilled me and still chills me even today. When she asked me where I was I told her that I was driving to a workshop in Cintsa, she asked me to stop the car. I knew there was a problem and her next words confirmed it. She said: "One of your male assistant nursing students has raped a patient.
I froze. "I am just giving you the heads up because the Daily Dispatch is going to phone you," she said before dropping the phone. I had to wake up from the nightmare and think of a response. I recalled what I had seen many a time on television which was mainly: "No Comment". However, newspapers have their own way of putting you on the spot. They started by telling me that they had learned that although

the students were training at Frere Hospital, they were actually being paid a monthly stipend by BIPH. This was true.

The next question was whether I knew about the rape at Frere Hospital and, thanks to the Matron, I confirmed. Then the usual question: "What is your comment". By now I had already decided what to say and I assured them that I would meet urgently with the board of the organisation and we would issue a statement the following day. Fortunately, we had a lawyer who represented the Newlands community who helped us to draft a response. I am not sure what happened to the student as he was arrested.

One of the best things that the Kellogg Foundation did was to ensure that the projects travelled to the countries where they were working. They always insisted on having myself and three representatives - one from the university or training institution, one from the health services and one from the community. Again, the communities had no problem in choosing their representative, however for the institutions it was always a struggle. We usually let them fight it out on their own until they decided and gave us the name. Through the project we travelled to West Virginia, Boston and Miami in the USA. We also went to Canada to McMaster and Sherbrook Universities, and as far afield as the Philippines.

The trip to McMaster University was aimed at enabling the South African delegation of 25 people to learn about problem-based learning. The outing to Niagara Fall was one of the highlights of the trip. In the Philippines we saw how primary health care facilities were growing medicinal plants that were used for treating some ailments that the patients presented with. We also went to Kenya and Egypt. I did not participate in all the trips, but whenever I travelled I made sure that I saw one or two other cities or countries. The extra leg of the trip was usually planned before leaving home and the ticket was arranged accordingly. When we went to Miami in the US, we planned with Gail Andrews, a director from a Kellogg Foundation project in the Western Cape, to spend three days in Disneyland in Orlando, Florida.

I was invited to the to the Salzburg Seminar in Austria, which was held at the Schloss Leopoldskron. Those of my age will remember the musical film "Sound of Music" which starred Julie Andrews. It was filmed in this castle on the Austrian side of the Alps. After the seminar, I want with another colleague, Neil Myburg, to the World Health Organization (WHO) in Geneva, Switzerland, and came home via Germany, at no extra charge to my ticket.

The visit to Kenya was slightly different. Many project staff and board members of the project, myself included, struggled with the concept of community participation in health. This was understandable, given our country's history where black people did not participate in any decisions that affected their lives. The Kenyan visit not only exposed us to health-care services that were managed and financed by community members but it also afforded us the opportunity to be trained by the African Medical and Research Foundation (AMREF) group on community-based health care. We visited beautiful places like Lake Nakuru and Lake Victoria which we could see every morning from our training location in Kisumu.

I was appointed to the advisory board of the University of Illinois in Chicago as they were also implementing community-based education for health personnel. I attended one-day meetings and I used this opportunity to see other places in the US. I visited friends in Boston after the meetings. At one stage I was invited to facilitate in a week's training programme of the US and South American projects. I could also invite friends and colleagues whose accommodation the University of Illinois Partnership would pay for as long as they could pay for their tickets. I was joined on this trip by the late Sis Nomathemba Ngani, Felicia Mazwi and my old friend Lulu Nkonzo-Mthembu.

I was invited to the Mexico Partnership after one of the University of Illinois meetings. After a 17-hour flight from home, I was exhausted but I still travelled from Chicago to Mexico for another five-day conference and visit to their community-based education (CBE) projects. I was to be joined by another South African from the BIPH project, Nonceba Mnyute.

When I finally left the polluted air of the streets of Mexico City and was resting in the hotel room, I heard somebody shouting my name in a familiar South African accent. Only to find that Nonceba was calling me. When I enquired why she had not asked the reception for my room number, she mentioned that they had told her but because of the Spanish accent she could not make out the number clearly and she could only understand the floor number. It was nice to have somebody from home to explore Mexico with and to visit the various CBE projects where their medical and nursing students were assigned. We also visited local tourist sites including the beautiful pyramids near Mexico City. Travel opens your horizons and enables you to relate to people from all walks of life.

CHAPTER 7

MANAGING PEOPLE IS NOT EASY

In addition to travel and exposure the BIPH project became my stepping stone to bigger projects and bigger organisations. I was recruited by the first project to work with the Department of Health, in 1997, the Equity Project. It was based in Bisho, the capital city of the newly established Eastern Cape Province.

The Equity Project was funded by the United States Agency for International Development (USAID) and was managed by a US-based company called Management Sciences for Health (MSH). It was the first US-funded project in the country, with a mind-boggling $50 million budget over a period of seven years.

I got onto the project with all the confidence of somebody who has been head hunted. My confidence soon disappeared. The Equity Project was huge with more than 30 staff members from six different countries - compared to the eight staff members of BIPH. Even with a good and thorough orientation,

I took time to fully understand the different programmes. All I knew was that it was supporting the Eastern Cape Department of Health (ECDOH).

Whilst trying to find my feet, I had to submit my first monthly report. I cannot remember what I wrote. All I can remember is that the report was reviewed by three people. It was marked with blue, red and black pens. What was interesting was the B/S on the margin that was written in the red pen. Confused, I asked Joan Littlefield, one of my American colleagues, what it meant. She laughed her lungs out as she explained that it meant "Bullshit". I was shocked, more so that it was the chief of party (director) who had written the comment, the one who had recruited me. Joan suggested that I go to him and ask for an explanation. That is when I got a full lecture of what the project was trying to do, what the different programmes were doing and how I fitted in in the whole puzzle. I also got a mentor for life in Dr Jon Rhode, the chief of party.

The Eastern Cape Department of Health (ECDOH) had the huge task of creating one health system from the many systems in the province, and to ensure a change from a curative service to a primary health care approach. The clinics, and not the hospital, were to be the first entry for people accessing the health-care system. Jon explained that one of the programmes in the project was to assist the province in developing a uniform set of information system for monitoring, evaluation and reporting on all health activities.

The lesson from the Kellogg Foundation visit came to mind but here the scope was a hundred times bigger. My role was to make sure that nurses throughout the province understood and used the health information system in their facilities and districts. Seeing that I was lost, Jon Rohde assured me that I would get all the training I needed to equip me for the role. This was done by sending me to the University of Western Cape's Winter School.

After attending the Advanced Course on the District Health Information System (DHIS), I felt confident enough to train nurses. I travelled to all the eight health districts in the province. The one week's training included a visit to a clinic for practical implementation of the information system. Many of the older nurses were not so enthusiastic about the programme and found the calculation of indicators to be a challenge. The young ones loved it and soon they were also training others.

The DHIS is one of the initiatives where I can say I participated in its development from scratch like the Community Based Education for Health Personnel, and they are both still being used. The DHIS is not only used throughout the country, but in other countries as well and has now evolved to an advanced electronic system.

The training, on-site mentoring and monitoring of implementation of the health information system took me to places that I never thought existed in the province, some of them shocked me. I had never travelled further than Butterworth in the east and Jeffreys Bay in the west. I found myself in places like Flagstaff, Qumbu, Mvenyane and a clinic in maybe one of the most remote areas of the province, namely Afsondering Clinic in the Maluti area in the Alfred Nzo District. I was shocked and reminded of Ghana when I saw places like Mount Frere. I also appreciated the vastness and rural nature of the province which makes it impossible to stick to the World Health Organization (WHO) guidelines of 5km to the nearest health facility.

The visits also gave me an opportunity to appreciate how much nurses in the province sacrifice to serve communities in remote and rural areas. Some of them have never been visited by a doctor. One of the many acts of kindness, which shows how nurses go out of their way to help their patients, is one I saw at Magadla Clinic. I visited the clinic on a very cold day in Maluti, which can be a very cold place because of the close Lesotho Mountains. I found one nurse and an assistant nurse with a waiting room full of patients. As I went to the offices with the nurse, we went past the maternity room where a patient was in labour. The nurses had heater on with a big pot of boiling water. The lid was open to allow the steam to warm the place for the woman and her soon-to-be delivered baby. They were working in a cold consulting room, having sacrificed the only heater in the clinic for the patient.

The Equity Project facilitated province-wide training in all its programmes and updated nurses on new treatment regimens, including the management of HIV/AIDS which was fast becoming a pandemic with no cure. Workshops were held in hotels for three to five days. This was always a highly prized opportunity by nurses, some of whom had never stayed in hotels before. The best workshops were those held in East London at the beachfront.

The project was a seven-year venture starting in the Eastern Cape in the first five years, with lessons learned and practices shared throughout the country in the sixth and seventh years.

I am one of those who had to facilitate the training and implementation of the health system throughout the country, having been one of its architects. This experience helped me to work in other counties like Uganda and Zimbabwe, assisting health professionals in implementing and using health information to monitor and evaluate their work.

In the sixth year, leadership of the project was taken over by a South African, Dr Thobile Mbengashe. He later moved to Pretoria to facilitated the countrywide expansion of the project. Jon Rhode was now a senior technical advisor to the project. MSH was looking for a deputy chief of party to lead the Eastern Cape team. There was a lot of speculation and jostling for the position. I did not consider myself to be in the competition as there were people who had started before me. I had joined the project three years after it had started. Also, the project had been led by male doctors beforehand.

In 2001, myself and two male colleagues were attending a USAID-sponsored senior executive programme. We attended four weeks of the programme at the University of Witwatersrand with two weeks held at Harvard University in Boston. Being the head office and based in Boston, MSH invited us to a party on the last day of the programme. During the party the President of MSH, Dr Ron O'Connor, whispered to me that they wanted me to be the deputy chief of party. This was said with a warning that I was not to share the information with anyone yet. I did not get a chance to be shocked until the following day when it hit me. I realised that the male doctors in the team, black and white, would be reporting to me who would be in a position that they also wanted and maybe felt entitled to.

I was told that the deputy directors name would be announced in the following staff meeting. Call me a coward or a strategist but I decided to honour an invitation from Abaqulusi District in KwaZulu-Natal for training on the health information system in that week. I did not want to see the faces of my colleagues when the announcement was made. As we were eager to roll out the health information system in the country, I was granted permission to be absent from the meeting. When I went back to the hotel in the evening I had so many calls from those who congratulated me. I noted those who did not call. A call from one of the female colleagues, Betty Ncanywa, explained it all. She told me that there was complete silence when the announcement was made, until she shouted "Viva Igama labafazi Viva" (Bravo to women). With her bold move, Betty broke the ice and also secured me support from all the female colleagues.

I had good working relations with most of the staff members. However, men - especially doctors - do not take kindly to being led by a female. Some instances and utterances I ignored. The one that got under my skin and made me really angry was a comment from one of the doctors. It was the time of performance reviews where I had to have one-on-one meetings with those that I directly supervised.

I was called by this colleague to a workshop that he was facilitating in East London. We met outside and I am not sure how the discussion went but all that I can remember are his words when he said: "You must remember, I am not used to being supervised by a black, female nurse." Although I was stunned, I reminded him that: "I have also never supervised a white, male doctor." It was only as I was driving to Bisho that the anger came back so overwhelmingly that I had to stop the car and calm myself. The following day, after I had calmed down, I set up an appointment with the doctor for us to continue with the performance review, during which I asked him what he would like me to do in order that we had smooth working relation. He requested that we have regular meetings, I suppose to get used to the idea of this black, female, nurse supervisor.

My appointment as the Deputy Chief of Party started my globetrotting again. I visited the head office in Boston several times. I was impressed and learned a lot from the work culture of my American colleagues. Those we worked with in South Africa would always remind us that the resources we were using were from the American taxpayers' money, a message that we could do with here at home.

CHAPTER 8

STAND UP FOR WHAT YOU WANT

When the Equity project came to an end in 2003, I was offered a position as a Principal Program Associate at the head office in Boston. I again left South Africa in the middle of summer on the 9th of January 2004 and arrived to deep snow in Boston, Massachusetts. I arrived at the MSH office at 11h00 and at 12 midday I was in a meeting, with my luggage. We were discussing a proposal to apply for funding for a project in Uganda, which defined my future participation in all proposals being developed for projects in Africa.

I was tired and drowsy during the meeting after a 17-hour trip and may not have been paying full attention, something that I regretted as I later had to work on the project in Uganda. The office had organised bed and breakfast accommodation where I was to stay until I found a permanent place. After I had dropped my luggage, I had to go out into the snow again to look for a shop to buy food for the evening and the following morning. Not only was Boston cold the people were cold, with the exception of some of those that I had met in South Africa when they visited the Equity Project. I was cold and lonely in the bed and breakfast place, with the owners coming only in the mornings. I asked myself the old question: "What the hell was I doing here?" It was not as if I did not have job offers at home.

MSH had two offices in their headquarters, one in Centre Street and one in Allendale Street. I was stationed in the one at Centre Street, Jamaica Plain. We were only three blacks in the office, all women. The one woman was a local elderly black American. She never said more than good morning to me. The other one was a young Nigerian woman, with whom I got along very well during and outside work. She assisted me in getting around to look for a place to stay.

Fortunately, another MSH employee who was going back home to the Philippines offered me his apartment in West Roxbury, with all that was in it in terms of furniture, pots and pans and even linen. He also sold me his car, which was a 1982 Toyota Corolla, which was still in a good condition. We agreed that I would send the money to him via the pouches that MSH regularly sent to the field offices. I only realised at the end of the month that, after I had received my bi-weekly payments, that I was going to struggle financially. When I signed the two-year contract from home the money looked good when converted to rands. My apartment cost me $1 500 which at the time translated to about R7 500. This was equal to the bond I was paying for my house at home, in Gonubie, in East London.

Pinky was still at the University of the Western Cape and she was using my car that I was still paying for. Money was the first and foremost reason why I renegaded on my two-year contract and left the US within six months. Also, I had thought that Pinky would be able to join me in the US and so get a chance of furthering her studies there. I leaned that because she was over 21 years of age she could not join me on my type of work permit.

I realised that my Filipino colleague had actually done me a favour by selling me his car as I had to take two buses from West Roxbury where I stayed to the office. However, I did not have the guts to get into the car and drive. The steering wheel was on the left and driving was on the wrong side compared to what I was used to at home. I decided to take a few driving lessons from a driving school, and eventually had the guts to drive myself to work. Even then, I would drive nicely when following other cars until I had to turn or get into a traffic circle, then I would get totally confused. Many a time, I would face oncoming traffic with the resultant hooting and shouting. I enjoyed the Sunday morning drives to the shops as there was less traffic.

Things improved when the weather improved around April. Friends started inviting me out. What I found strange, as a South African, was people inviting you to a restaurant whereas I had invited them to my house. I had even had parties for them at home. Of course, a couple took me to their home. One friend in particular, Mary O'Neil, invited me on a weekend trip at her holiday home in Cape Cod. Together with Maria Pia, another friend, we spent a lovely time at the beach and site seeing. We visited the area where the homestead of the Kennedy family, the home of the late President JF Kennedy, is situated.

At work, things were not bad at all. I soon learned the routine of asking for the code of each project I worked on so as to charge my time against that project. I visited our third office in Washington DC to make a presentation on the Equity Project. I was pleasantly surprised when, on greeting one black American young girl, she immediately identified my accent as being South African. It turned out that she had spent a year in Cape Town as an exchange student at the University of Cape Town. She took it upon herself to point out all there was to see in Washington DC, including the White House. What I enjoyed most were the Washington and Lincoln Memorial Museums. What touched me most was the Holocaust Memorial Museums, where - similar to the Hector Peterson Memorial - one is able to watch a 13-minute film on how the Jews were murdered by the Germans during the Second World War.

Another friend who invited me to her place insisted that I should drive to her house. I made it safely to her place, using directions that she had sent. However, driving back home I got lost and found myself driving around for four hours before I somehow recognised my street and my apartment block.

As the months went by my financial situation got worse. What made the situation worse was the two different taxes that were deducted from my salary, the federal and state taxes. Also, in the US, there is no 13th cheque (bonus) like we have at home. I decided it was time to leave the US and go back home where my salary was much better than at head office. I realised that you actually earned more money when you are in the field, which explained why Americans tend to visit field offices. Using dollars, they can stay at places that are cheaper than in the US. They also don't pay as much for food and other commodities. They use very little of the travel allowance or the per diem as it is called. From travelling a couple of times to the project in Uganda, I also made some extra money, however, this was not a constant extra.

In taking action about my financial situation, I requested a meeting with the president of the organisation, Ron. Meetings typically took place in a restaurant. Ron and I were comfortable with each other from the time of him choosing me to be the deputy chief of party of the Equity Project, to recruiting me to head office. This is one thing that I appreciate about working for NGOs. There are less barriers to talking to the powers that be than in government where, whatever you want to discuss with a senior person, your immediate supervisor has to know about. I explained to Ron that I had not come to the US to be poor. I wanted to go back home or even go to Afghanistan as MSH had just won a five-year contract in that country. So long as I left the US. Ron was very understanding and although there was no post in the current project in South Africa, he would look around for a post in a field project. By June 2004, MSH had won the contract for the project in Uganda and I was appointed technical advisor to the project and was on a flight to Uganda on the 30th of June 2004 with my furniture to follow.

Before leaving the US, I made a trip to New York. How do you stay in the US and not spend time in this famous city? I had a good reason to visit. My uncle, Bidwell Nkomo, had asked me to look up his son, Botshabelo (Bushy). To my uncle Boston and New York were close to each other as long as you were in the same country. Bushy Nkomo, my cousin, had left home in Lady Frere in 1977 with uncle Aubrey Nkomo. For more than 30 years he had never come home, although he was in contact with his family and phoned them regularly. Having not seen him for such a long time, we had to tell each what we would be wearing so that we could identify each other when I arrived at the bus station in New York.

We met and took a train to Harlem where he stayed. I was fascinated by the place and we sat outside till late in the night. He was eager to hear everything about home and his family. He did not understand all the new names like, Chris Hani District and Emalahleni Local Municipality, where his former home in Lady Frere was. He was excited to be with somebody from home and speaking isiXhosa.

Everything looks glamourous when you visit a place until you stay in it and see the good and the bad, the beautiful and the ugly. The glamour of working in the United States of America was what enticed me when I was offered an opportunity to go and work at head office in Boston. However, within six months it was just unbearable. I did not stay and use my two-year working permit.

CHAPTER 9

RESPONSIBILITY AND ACCOUNTABILITY ARE PART OF OUR TRAINING

I first visited Uganda in May 2004 before moving there permanently. The May visit coincided with Brenda Fassie's death. To the Ugandans it was as if they had lost their own sister. Getting out of Entebbe Airport and all the way to my hotel in Kampala Brenda's music was blaring from all corners. I even got condolences when they learned that I was from South Africa.

On the 1st of July 2004, deployed by MSH, I got to my working station at the Inter Religious Council of Uganda (IRCU). The first thing that struck me was that all the staff members, with the exception of the receptionist and cleaner, were men. During the welcome meeting they openly expressed that they wished that MSH had sent a male technical advisor.

IRCU is an organisation made up of all the major denominations in the country, namely: the Roman Catholic Church (RCC), the Church of the Province of Uganda (Church of Uganda-COU), the Uganda Orthodox Church (UOC), the Uganda Muslim Supreme Council (UMSC), the Seventh-Day

Adventist Uganda Union (SDAUU), the Born-Again Faith in Uganda (BAF) and the National Alliance of Pentecostal and Evangelical Churches in Uganda (NAPECU). I used to sit with Bishops and Muftis during the board meetings. They were mostly males, with one female, a member of parliament.

One of the staff members was a Muslim whose behaviour always caught me off guard. As they were all visiting the projects we decided to have our meetings on Fridays. Just before 1pm the guy would stand up, in the middle of the meeting, and announce that he was going to the Masque to pray. This was the first time I had come across something like this and I did not know how to handle it although it did not seem to bother his other colleagues.

The churches were all managing health facilities ranging from hospitals to primary health care clinics, as well as HIV/AIDS and Orphans and Vulnerable Children's programmes, which were spread throughout the country. My role was to assess those that qualified to receive funding from USAID, which was managed by MSH. I worked with a financial technical advisor, Silas, who was based in Kenya. I used MSH's assessment tool called the Management, Organisational and Sustainability Tool (MOST). I trained two staff members who were going to work on the organisational assessment and Silas trained the other two on financial assessment. We then got a list of all the health facilities to be assessed from the board members who represented all the churches.

In assessing the health facilities, we travelled the length and breadth of Uganda. We undertook the first trip to the western region, in Mbarara District, on a Sunday afternoon. We stopped for lunch along the way where I asked to use the bathroom. I was shocked to find that the toilet was a hole on the floor. I struggled to use it. I came back and told the guys that wherever we were going to sleep, in the bed and breakfast places, they must first check the toilets and if it was not the type I am used to, we were not going to sleep there. This they duly did. One of the most enjoyable visits was to a facility in Jinja, which is a beautiful waterfall and the source of the Nile River. We had gone there on a Friday and spent the Saturday along the lake. I also took Pinky, Thuli and my grandson Hope to Jinja when they came to visit me in Uganda.

I visited the local USAID office regularly as I was also tasked with helping the Uganda AIDS Commission (UAC) in the implementation of their mid-term review and revision of the National HIV/AIDS Strategic Framework, amongst other things. I nearly fought with the young American girl who was the project contact person in the country. I had said that I admire the work culture of Americans, but some of them can be really arrogant. When I left the USAID office, I was so angry that instead of calling for a taxi, I decided to walk back to the office. Along the way I saw the South African High Commissioners Office. I had not bothered to report myself there before but on this day, I went in and informed the receptionist that I wanted to be known that I was in the country. I told them that I might assault somebody and if that happened, I would like the commissioner to bail me out. The office staff were shocked as Ugandans are normally calm and peaceful people. They called a South African man who worked in the office, who laughed at my story. He remarked that he missed that about South Africa where people spoke their mind when they were upset. I had found myself a friend from home.

My financial and emotional situation improved dramatically in Uganda. To start with I was paid in dollars in a country whose currency was 746 Ugandan Shillings to the dollar at the time. Secondly, I had an allowance called third country national, which I did not know about. Thirdly, the organisation paid for my accommodation. Also, my dollar salary was untaxed. I tried in vain to register for tax in Uganda, but it just did not materialise until I left for home. Lastly, I was only four hours from home which meant I could visit my family more frequently.

We were running a workshop for all the project grantees. I was orientating them on a monitoring and reporting system that I had developed with the help of Calle Hedberg from the Health Information System Programme (HISP). The aim was to make reporting easier and more regular. During lunchtime I received a call that really surprised me. It was from a Ugandan number but his first word was such a lovely surprised. He said 'Mankomo where are you?" The mention of my clan name in Uganda gave me such joy. I recognised the voice immediately as that of Prince Zolile Ncamashe, an old friend. I could not wait for the workshop to finish so that I could catch up with him. He was with a delegation from the Eastern Cape (Amathole District). They were hosted by the Ugandan government to learn more about their HIV/AIDS programmes. It turned out he was with Nkosi Langa Mavuso and Sakhumzi Somyo. My friend, Ntsoaki Sepoko, who was working at the Department of Foreign Affairs in Kenya, was coming to visit me in Uganda on the same weekend. We had a typical South African party.

We had visited more than 20 projects and were left with one that was in Arua District in the northern part of Uganda. I did not understand the reluctance of my male colleagues in going to Arua. I asked Sarah, a local girl from another USAID-funded project who I had befriended. She told me that Arua was where the Lord's Resistance Army (LRA) was located and there was still a lot of attacks on the locals by the army. The matter was raised in a board meeting, with the Roman Catholic Church representative complaining that their health services in Arua were suffering because of a lack of funds. My male colleagues pointed out that I was the technical advisor and therefore I was to go.

It was November and Pinky, Thuli and my grandson Hope were visiting me in Uganda. I think the entrenched culture of nursing, of taking responsibility, is what made me take the risk. The youngest staff member in the organisation, who was responsible for finance, offered to travel with me. We were to fly from Entebbe to Aura. I did not realise that we were going to fly in a small 12-seater plane. What was worse, there was no airport at Arua. We landed on a small landing strip where the plane felt like a car travelling on a gravel road. We were picked up by the project staff and drove to their health facility which was a beautiful clinic.

Along the way we saw several groups of people in enclosed spaces. I was told that these were camps for internally displaced people (IDPs). Not far from the small township there was a forest and I was told that the LRA solders were camped out there. The facility, like most Roman Catholic health facilities, was well run. What impressed me most was their data management, monitoring and evaluation as demonstrated by the graphs on the wall. The HIV incidence and prevalence were almost five times higher than anywhere in the country. According to the staff, this was due to the fact that women and young girls in the area were regularly raped by the solders of the LRA.

Despite anxieties and fears, my nursing training enabled me to block out everything and focus on the HIV/AIDS programme. We conducted and finished the assessment on the same day but there was no flight back to Kampala until the following day. We spent the night at a highly guarded and heavily secured accommodation. The following morning, from 8 am there was no network. We were told that some government officials were visiting the area and the networks had to be off so that the LRA would not know the whereabouts of the government officials. I was relieved to land at Entebbe Airport and be reunited with my family.

I enjoyed Uganda as the people are friendly and - like many of us - when we see a black person, we assume they are locals. Many a time people spoke to me in Buganda, which is the local language. This happened so much that I had to learn a few words, and I am now able to greet and ask people how they are in the Buganda language.

My apartment had a beautiful view of the Ugandan side of Lake Victoria. I was also not affected by load shedding which I saw for the first time in Uganda. This was because I was staying in an area where mostly the diplomats stayed. I boasted that we do not have such a thing at home, little did I know that it was going to be an almost daily occurrence from 2010. I had a driver throughout my stay in Uganda. I just could not drive in the streets where you will find three cars going in the same direction in a lane meant for only one car. Added to the chaos was the Boda Bodas (or motorcycles) that are a form of public transport. The only time the streets were empty was when President Museveni was travelling with his long convoy that even included an ambulance.

I grew closer to the only female board member, the member of parliament. She shared with me how they usually took money in bags when going to canvas for votes. This was called "shaking the tree" and locals were so used to it that they would tell the politician that so and so who came before you shook the tree much better, meaning that they gave more money than you were giving. I learned a lot about African politics.

I came home for the December holidays and felt the pull of home and being with my family, however I went back in January 2005. We went on another travelling experience to evaluate progress in the health establishments that we had funded. I continued strengthening the use of the health information system.

I was recruited by Health Systems Trust (HST). I was interviewed telephonically in January 2005 and although the salary was going to be less than what I was earning in Uganda, I accepted as the idea of going back home was appealing. I had the task of reporting this to my immediate supervisor who told me in no uncertain terms that MSH had taken me from South Africa to Boston and from Boston to Uganda and were not about to let me go without finishing my contract. Again, my saviour, Ron, came up with the suggestion that if I wanted to go back home I should actually work in the project that MSH had at the time in Pretoria, South Africa.

This was a pleasant and welcome offer as Pinky had just started her internship with the Department of the Water Affairs in Pretoria. We were going to be staying together again as a family. It also meant that I would spend my December holidays with my aged parents, my siblings, family and friends. The experience of all the places I had travelled thus far made me appreciate my family even more.

CHAPTER 10

THE NURSING PROFESSION OPENS MANY DOORS

I joined MSH's Integrated Primary Health Care (IPHC) project in June 2005. I worked with my former Chief of Party, Dr Thobile Mbengashe, and a few of the support staff who had moved to Pretoria. The project was now working in eight districts in five provinces, namely, the Eastern Cape, (Alfred Nzo and Chris Hani districts), KwaZulu-Natal (Harry Gwala and uThungulu districts), Mpumalanga (Gert Sibande District), Limpopo (Capricorn and Sekhukhune districts) and the North West (Bojanala District).

I started as a technical advisor working on the orphans and vulnerable children (OVC) programme. We were developing a programme to fund the organisation that supported the OVCs. I was travelling again, but the beauty of it this time was that at the end of the trip I joined my family and could spend time with my grandson Hope. One important lesson that I learned in working with OVCs was taught to me by one of their staff members. On completion of a visit to her orphanage, and after the children had sung for us, she asked us to hug the kids. From the way they clung during those hugs, one understood how they missed that simple human touch that we – as well as our own children and grandchildren - take for granted.

IPHC was also implementing a number of other programmes including Strengthening of Primary Health Care (PHC) Services, District Development, Maternal and Child Health, a youth programme and the OVC programme. The project had very good and competent people who were based in the different provinces and came to Pretoria quarterly for staff meetings. It is within the project that we initiated and institutionalised the programme reviews by the districts where we were working. We championed PHC reviews which are now conducted routinely in most health district. We also institutionalised the use of the District Health Information System (DHIS) in the review of programmes. Ntuthu Dlamini became our roving trainer on the DHIS.

MSH advertised the post of a Deputy to Dr Mbengashe. I applied and got the position. As a deputy chief of party, I was responsible for all the programmes. The first thing that I changed was the reporting. There seemed to be a competition, with the technical advisers working in the same province, in the presentation of their work. It got to a point where I heard that four staff members visited Nomponjwana Clinic in the uThungulu District, in KwaZulu Natal, in four cars. Each one was coming for his or her programme. Imagine how intimidated the nurses in that facility felt. I asked all the staff in a province to work as a team. They were to sit together, plan their activities for the month and - where possible - travel together. Most importantly, they were to sit together and prepare a provincial report which was to be presented by one person from each province.

Managing people is not easy, especially when they are scattered in five provinces. I discovered this in two instances. We had a support visit by our project manager from MSH in Boston. We decided to take her to visit some of our growth monitoring sites in the North West. The technical advisor, who had reported many visits to the facilities and reported on the activities, did not know where the facilities were. She kept stopping and asking for directions. Imagine my embarrassment and anger!

The second instance was when we were going to have a workshop in Mpumalanga. We asked the technical advisors to get three quotations as per the policy. I was surprised when the financial manager showed me the three quotes. She had noticed that the font and font size were the same, even the spelling mistakes made were in the same words on all three. Of course, the advisor denied any knowledge of the whole thing.

Dr Mbengashe left MSH a few months after I had been appointed as a deputy chief of party. MSH summoned me to Boston. I was told in no uncertain terms that they did not doubt my technical skills; however, they were worried about my management and leadership skills. They decided to take a chance on me on condition that I got a mentor to mentor me in the skills that they felt I lacked. They promoted me to the chief of party position but I was to go home and look for the mentor. This is one area that the public sector can learn from.

Many good technical people are promoted to management positions because of their technical skills, they may fall short in leadership and management skills. Had those employees had somebody to mentor them in management and leadership, they would have excelled. When I raised this issue with a group of senior government managers, the response was that when you are employed in a senior position in government, it is assumed that you are good. I am not sure about this - it is open for discussion.

I found one of the best strategists as a mentor. Lenard Smith had worked as a turnaround strategist in many companies, organisations and institutions. We met for three days in a week, every month, for six months. MSH paid for this mentoring. He started with simple things like time management and running meetings and then progressed to more complex areas like conflict management. Each time he would leave me with an example of a work-related problem to solve which we would discuss in our next meeting. He also became my springboard to bounce new ideas and challenges off. I learned a lot from my mentor, with the most important lesson being that you cannot manage alone. As a manager you have to build a team as well as work through and with people

I encountered one of my old problems: a white male (not a doctor this time) who was an accountant. Gerhard Combrink was the best of the five candidates that we interviewed for the position of a financial director. I had to ask during the interview, when it was clear that he was the one best suited for the position: "How would you feel being supervised by a black female?" Of course, he stated that he had no problems, which turned out to be true. He was good at his job, respectful and a pleasure to work with.

The project had to expand as we were venturing into supporting the district with the Anti-Retroviral Treatment roll out. I had to recruit doctors as the Nurses Initiated Management of Anti-Retroviral Therapy (NIMART) programme had not started yet. The one advantage of an international organisation is that you are able to attract the best people from any country. We ended up with two doctors, one from Zambia and one from Nigeria. In the Eastern Cape I was fortunate to get a local person who was good at the programme, Dr Nozipho Jaxa. The programme for the OVC was later managed by somebody from Zimbabwe. As mentioned before, with the exception of a couple staff members I had a good team that delivered measurable results.

In 2009, I received an email inviting me to apply to be a member of the Technical Review Panel (TRP) member of the Global Fund to Fight AIDS, Tuberculosis and Malaria. I was excited and worked on their long application form, although I was not clear what the work entailed. I did not expect to be called to Geneva in the same year. When I received the invitation to attend the two-week meeting, I had to request for permission from MSH. My employer was only too excited to have their own employee at this global forum. The TRP team was huge and had more than 30 people from all over the world. There were two South African, white male doctors with a typical attitude. I knew both of them from home, but one still had the audacity to ask me how I had got into the Global Fund. Hardened by now, I simply asked him if the Global Fund was a reserve of White Male Doctors and - at any rate - even if it was, I, a black, female nurse, had qualified to be there and can do whatever they were able to do.

The first time at a Global Fund Meeting made me realise that we were actually disbursing billions of dollars to countries all over the world. The work was heavy, with three proposals to go through every night that were to be presented the following day. The document not only included the actual proposal but the strategic plans of those countries and huge budgets. We worked as teams of three and each one had to take the lead in presenting a country and the recommendations to fund or no to fund it. I reviewed proposals from countries that I heard never heard about before, like Suriname.

The beauty about the Global Fund Meetings was that you travelled first class. You also planned your own trip. I planned it in such a way that I went via London, Saudi Arabia and even Addis Ababa. The Global Fund Meetings were held on either side of Lake Geneva, either the Switzerland or the French side. On some of my trips to Boston or Geneva I went through the Netherlands to visit Pinky, who was studying for her masters degree at Maastricht University. It is during these visits to her that mother and daughter went to the red-light district in Amsterdam.

One of the lessons I learned during my time as a leader and manager at MSH project was the importance of reading all documents, especially the reports. I would sit outside in summer on Saturdays and Sundays, at my home in Pretoria, and read every report submitted quarterly by the technical advisors and field staff. This is how I discovered that some of them actually copied and pasted from the previous quarter's report. I supposed that was done thinking that I would not notice it. Unfortunately for them, discovering this only made me read even more.

The second lesson was to document all meetings and exchanges with staff. Twice, I was reported to the head office in Boston by some staff members who were unhappy about one thing or another, or my management style. MSH instituted an inquiry and I was exonerated by the written evidence that I produced to show how I had handled the issues they were unhappy about.

In 2010, after more than fifteen years in management positions, I got tired. The work was just no longer challenging me anymore. Also, Pinky had decided to go back to Cape Town. She was not coping with the Pretoria weather as she is prone to allergies. She took my grandson, Hope with her. I found myself alone in Pretoria, with a sprinkling of friends. Thirdly, MSH had employed a very capable and very intelligent deputy chief of party, Dr Tracey Naledi. She was a breath of fresh air to the project. Her enthusiasm and easy-going manner made me realise that I had in fact instituted a succession plan and it was time for me to move on.

I decided to go into consulting. The important thing was to be with Pinky and Hope in Cape Town. I had offers to consult from two companies. The Health Information Systems Programme (HISP) wanted me to support their USAID-funded project in Zimbabwe. The Zimbabwe Ministry of Health and Child Care was reviving its health Information System called ZimHISP. I was travelling from Cape Town to Zimbabwe every month, staying for a week. I travelled the length and breadth of Zimbabwe visiting health facilities to provide on-site support for nurses on the information system. I also attended planning and programme review meetings. I travelled from Harare to Bulawayo and even to smaller towns like Mukoni, Mazowe, Bindura, Rusape and even spent time at the township of

Marondera in Harare. I also had the opportunity to go to the Victoria Falls, which I found more beautiful and natural compared to Niagara Falls.

The second assignment was with Health Partners International in Botswana. I was working with the Ministry of Health and Wellness of Botswana. I supported the Directorate of Health Inspectorate in developing their strategic plan as they were being established as an independent unit. I spent the first week of the month in Zimbabwe and the second week in Botswana. When the Botswana project ended, HISP employed me permanently and added another project where I supported OR Tambo District in the Eastern Cape, the Gert Sibande District in Mpumalanga and Pretoria in Gauteng, in the development of the HIV/ AIDS information system. I had one week in which to write reports. The travelling was taxing, and the only consolation was being with my family over the weekends and the one week of report-writing.

I still attended Global Fund Meetings whenever requested. In 2012, on the 22nd of June, I celebrated my 60th birthday with over 30 people from all corners of world and singing happy birthday for me in Geneva. I reflected on the fact that I had spent my 40th birthday in Ghana, my 52nd birthday in Boston, in the US and my 60th birthday in Geneva in Switzerland. My nursing profession had made all this possible. At home Pinky had organised a birthday at Terra Gonna Lodge, in Hout Bay, Cape Town.

2012 is also the year the year Pinky got married and I had my second grandson, Aidan, Lizo. I realised that I could not stay with her and her husband as they were newlyweds and needed their space. Also, I had very few friends in Cape Town. It is not easy to make new friends after 60. My friends were in the Eastern Cape and I was on my way home.

CHAPTER 11
WORKING FOR THE NEW GOVERNMENT FOR THE FIRST TIME—AN EYE OPENER

In 2013, I resigned from HISP to start a TBHIV project in Duncan Village, East London. I was back in time, to the old streets I had driven through when I was working on my first community health project in the geriatric programme. The place was still the same but the disease challenges were different. I worked with young women who were providing Directly Observed TB Support (DOTS) to people with TB. They were also referring them to the local clinics for HIV testing. It was during this time that I got a position with the Eastern Cape Department of Health as a director for monitoring and evaluation.

I started in the Department of Health on the 1st of September 2014. On the 17th of September, whilst sitting in my car during lunch time, I got a call from somebody from the Office of the

Premier. The call went like this: "Mrs Mazaleni the MPAT report is due today." My response was typical of a layman. I asked "What is the MPAT report?" The person on the line must have been shocked at my question as her next statement was that it is a report that is submitted by the Monitoring and Evaluation Directorate of which I was the director. Realising that the person was not about to give me a lecture on this MPAT report, I promised to call her back.

I rushed to my office and asked the staff about this MPAT. Only one of them knew what it was. I heard for the first time that it was a Management Performance Assessment Tool, that each government department submitted to the National Department of Performance Monitoring and Evaluation (DPME). Getting my hands on the document was a struggle as passwords are used to gain access to it and I did not have one. I still admire my team about the way they rallied and ran around to get me a password.

When I saw the information required I realised that it needed months to collect, collate and load into the system. We did what we could and I finally drove back from Bisho to East London at 8pm. I knew what we submitted was sub-standard and resolved to make sure that the following year's report would definitely be better.

The reason I found myself in this predicament was due to a number of reasons. I joined the Department of Health for the first time in 2017 after working for more than 30 years in the health sector, most of which in public health in the non-governmental sector. I felt privileged to join the department at the ripe age of 62 years. I had gathered a lot of experience locally having trained at Frere Hospital in East London and working there before working as a lecturer in the province and later as a community health nurse in the rural areas in the province.

I had also worked nationally, supporting five of the eight provinces. Outside the country I had worked in Botswana, Uganda and Zimbabwe providing support to an MSH project in Nigeria and the United States of America. Coming back home to the Eastern Cape I saw the advert for a Director for Monitoring and Evaluation and realized that with my experience, I could actually contribute a lot to the province. I was called for the interview in July 2014. The panel that interviewed me was made up of three male doctors from the health department and one female from the Office of The Premier (OTP). I must have performed well in the interview because I was offered the position.

The Monitoring and Evaluation Department falls under the Strategy and Organisational Performance Directorate, which is also known as SOP. Between my appointment and starting work, I had one meeting with the head of SOP where he told me that he would not be around when I started in September as he was going on retirement. He gave me a brief description of the directorate and what its role was in the health department. He also gave me some reports. I tried to read these but could only understand the health language and not the structure of the reports, which made no sense to me. The fact that there were eight programmes was puzzling. I told myself that I would ask for an explanation of this during the orientation. Unfortunately, there was no orientation planned for me. This also raises the question as to whether the department thinks of, or has, any succession plans for key positions.

I was warmly welcomed by my three staff members on the day I started working. They showed me my office, which was a big room with a long table and chairs in the middle. Little did I know that we would spend long hours around that table and bond around it until we were a closely-knit family. After settling in, I sat down with my team and they gave me a run-down of what they were doing in the directorate. The male assistant director seemed to know more than the other two females one who was a nurse and the other a health technologist. They said that the gentleman was the one who worked closer with the chief director who was also a man. That was all I got in the form of orientation. I had to get used to the different reports and reporting schedules of the Treasury, National Department of Health (NDOH) Standing Committee on Health, MPAT and other unscheduled reports.

My team was great in terms of the structure and due dates and all the requirements for submission of the reports but not with the content. I spent my weekends reading the draft reports. I realised that the content did not tell me much and started wondering who these were written by and how these were written. Logic told me that the people who were in charge of the programmes were the ones who were supposed to write the narrative part of the reports. Many managers submitted the reports so late that to ask them to redo or explain what they had written would mean that the department would report late at the various institutions where the reports were to be submitted. I had to make sure that this did not continue. I realise that I would just have to put my foot down and demand reports from all those who were supposed to submit them.

These reports are actually required by law and the dates for submission are fixed with the submission schedule provided at the beginning of the year by the National Department of Health and Treasury. There was no way that I was going to fail to submit and I was not going to be late for submission. Having worked for United States Agency for International Development (USAID)-funded projects, I knew the meaning of accountability when implementing a programme. I phoned the programme managers at any time of the day and demanded the reports My staff were shocked by my approach, to which I replied that I was "old and ugly enough" not to be sacred of anybody. I was not doing what I did for myself but for the Department of Health. I recalled what a specialist said to a houseman when the records of the patients, like X-rays and blood results were not available. He said: "When you demand these results from the nurses, you will be unpopular for some time, but in the end, they will respect you."

What was a culture shock for me in the report-writing process was when a manager could not email a report? I kept on phoning her and got promises that it was on the way. Little did I know that this was literal, until a young man who claimed to be the manager's secretary walked in with a memory stick on which the report was saved so that it could be transferred onto my computer. I thought that this was a network problem, but later discovered that both the manager and the secretary did not know how to attach and email the report. This was unbelievable to somebody who worked for USAID-funded projects in Zimbabwe, Uganda and the USA. How on earth would I have sent reports to head office in the US if it was not by email? It said a lot about the recruitment, orientation and skills development in the department.

The reports were not only late but some had glaring grammatical and spelling mistakes and even content that did not explain the quantitative results. They were clearly written in a hurry. It seemed that managers did not make report-writing a priority, which begs the question of how can you work and not account for the resources that you are using in your work.

To correct this, I did it in my own style. During a quarterly review meeting - that is usually attended by all the top management members, district managers, the Head of Department and the Member of the Executive (MEC) - I flagged the exact responses that I had received on the screen. The embarrassment earned me a lot of enemies as people saw their work in front of them being shared with their colleagues and even district staff. After that, the quality of the reports improved as no one wanted to see his or her mistakes glaring at all the managers of the province.

The last straw in the lack of orientation in the directorate was when somebody from the Auditor General's (AG) office phoned me for an appointment. I had no idea of the role that the directorate played in the auditing process. The meeting was an eye opener. Apparently, we were supposed to submit the annual report for auditing where they compared what was planned in the Annual Performance Plan and the report.

Planning is done by another team in the directorate who were experienced in the process and therefore no problems were identified. Where we had an uphill battle was when the annual report was audited. Managers had to provide supporting documents and a portfolio of evidence in the area where they had performed well against the achieved indicators and also evidence of what they had done in areas where the targets were not met. We had to run after them again to get this evidence. The process improved the quality of our report as we knew that the AG was reading each and every line.

Confronted with the many challenges in the directorate, I had to develop a strategy to make our work easier. The first strategy was to get all three staff members on board. I started by training my staff on all the performance indicators that we were dealing with in terms of the numerator the denominator and what each indicator measured, what the expected performance was and what the minimum and maximum achievements meant. I divided the programmes amongst ourselves. When those who were not nurses felt insecure, I assured them that I was there as their resource and anybody can learn if they are willing to do so. I assured them that we were not dealing with rocket science but ordinary health issues that they were actually familiar with. Most importantly, I assured them that I would mentor them throughout the process until they felt confident.

We started the ritual of sitting around the table every time we had a draft report. We would look at it on the screen from the data projector and read it line by line. Human beings are wonderful people if you believe in them. By the time we were doing the exercise for the third time they were able to identify mistakes and question statements that were not clear. I usually bought lunch for all of us as this meant working late in order to meet the deadlines.

By the second year we had two additional deputy directors which lightened the burden of the number of programmes for each individual. They soon learned and appreciated the value of teamwork in the unit. By the time I left the department I had a well-oiled machine of people who knew exactly how to compile the reports and follow up all the necessary steps until the report was submitted on time to the right authority.
I encouraged my team to attend district performance review meetings. The picture you get at provincial level is somewhat different from what is happening at the lower levels. Attending the review meetings also broadened their outlook and gave myself and the team a deeper insight into the work done at district level.

The time of the dreaded MPAT report came again. This time all my staff members attended orientation meetings that were organised by the Office of the Premier (OTP). We all studied what evidence was needed and how it was to be loaded onto the system. I realised that to get good results I had to sit with all the units that were supposed to report and submit policies. We went through each requirement and got a key person in each unit who would load the information. The results for the second year I was in the department went from zero to three out of five. We already knew how we would improve in the following year. Throughout the following three years the score remained at four out of five.

I learned a lot about government legislation and processes from my role as the director of monitoring, evaluation and reporting. I still wonder if it would have been easier if there was an orientation programme that included all the processes, requirements and deadlines, or if the trial and error actually helped me. Maybe if I had been in the department before I would had fared better although I doubt this as directorates tend to work in silos in the department. The implementation of an orientation programme would be ideal at district and facility management level as well.

I have come across operational mangers who are promoted and have to be suddenly in charge of their colleagues. Many do not have any training on leadership and management. Problems arise when they have to discipline or point out poor performance of those that they supervise. They are not equipped to deal with these challenges as they did not have any orientation on the human resources and legal guidelines they learned these by trial and error.

CHAPTER 12

IT IS STILL A MAN'S WORLD

This chapter was written on the 9th of August 2020, on Women's Day in South Africa. Julius Malema has just made a statement at Mama Winnie Mandela's graveside. He said: "It is a man who decide which woman holds which position." This is true in health even though female nurses outnumber other health professionals. It is a man's world. This I experienced in the department of health. I acted as the head (Chief Director) of the Strategy and Organisational Performance Directorate for more than six months before the position was advertised. Automatically, I applied and was short listed. The panel consisted of two men and one woman. There were three candidates. The one candidate was a woman who had worked in the Monitoring and Evaluation Directorate. I was surprised by the third male candidate. He had flown in from Pretoria that morning. This was somebody who I had not only worked with but had supervised as a deputy chief of party in one of the USAID projects in the province.

The results of the interviews were even more surprising. He got the post. This was somebody who did not have a health background although he had ample experience in monitoring and evaluating health programmes. Not only was I a nurse with experience in monitoring and evaluation, but I also hold a masters degree in community health. He did not have a masters degree. I went into the interview confident and thought that I had answered all the questions in the right way. But the one thing that made me confident was the fact that I was already acting in the position and knew what the work entailed and how the directorate worked.

I am not sure if it was my age that put me at a disadvantage or not. However, if that was the consideration that swayed the panel, it did not work as the guy left a month after I had retired. The female deputy director general who was on the panel called me to her office to give me the letter that notified me that I had not been successful in my application. I could see that she was somewhat embarrassed, after all she could have sent the letter with a messenger.

I am human and it was natural for me to be angry and resentful. Thinking of my own experience, here was somebody else who had also never worked in government, let alone the monitoring, evaluation and reporting directorate with all its legal requirements. Here was someone I had supervised before, now in charge of me. Do I let him sink or swim like I did? I fell back on my old saying that "I am old and ugly enough not sink to that level". However, the relationship was not smooth sailing, I think whenever we disagreed we each thought about where we had come from and how we found ourselves on opposite sides of the table. However, we were also professionally enough to make the relationship work. To his credit, he organised a big retirement farewell party for me during my last provincial meeting.

Before handing over to my boss, I had ensured that the two vacant deputy directors posts in the unit were filled. In my ignorance of the system I asked around on how a panel was constituted and was told that for a deputy director's post you had to have directors in your panel. I asked two females and two male directors to be in the panel. Women can let you down sometimes and the two females I had asked pulled out of the panel on the morning of the interviews. The two males were available and indicated that I had to invite a member of the unions who turned out to be a man. The conclusion as you can guess - a man was appointed. For the second deputy director's interview I literally begged the women to participate and they did. Although we again appointed a man I felt the process was directed by the merits of the candidates. I also felt there was a balance in the unit as there were now three men and three women.

The appointment system at district level was, and should be, different as the leadership and management at this level is predominantly female. However, the process is not entirely without flaws. The most manipulated appointments are those of the lower level especially the data capturer. A matric certificate and computer literacy are all that is required for this position. With high unemployment rate amongst the youth, a data capturer's post can attract hundreds of applicants, some with masters degrees. However, this is where sons, daughters, nephews and nieces of those in management get to be appointed. In some instances, the children and relatives of the managers are employed in areas where they do not reside, with local young people overlooked.
As long as there was a position in a clinic or hospital, the managers, who are the first to know about these, would phone the managers in those areas for their preferred candidates. This would be agreed upon on condition that the person

returned the favour when they had a position in their districts in the future.

One feels sorry for all those unknown candidates who go to great lengths photocopying Identity documents (ID) and certificates, certifying them and submitting, hoping for employment, which never comes. Navigating the employment and appointment system in government is complex. More needs to be done before nurses are blamed. Though there are bad apples amongst nurses, there are a lot of good and hardworking individual, some of whom become demotivated by the appointments made and the lack of support.

CHAPTER 13
REWIRED NOT RETIRED

I left the Department of Health on the 30th of September 2017, and on the 1st of October 2017 I was employed, as a consultant, by a Cape Town-based company called Strategic Evaluation, Advisory and Development (SEAD). I was supporting the Amathole District with planning, monitoring and evaluation. I had not left the health sector after all. When I worked with the Department of Health in Bisho, I had moved back to my rural home in Krwakrwa in Alice. The distance from Alice to Bisho is more or less the same as the distance from Bisho to East London. However, in supporting the Amathole District I had to move back to East London. I stayed with one of my friends during the week and travelled to the village every weekend.

The contract with SEAD was for one year. However, as is the nature of projects, the funding cycle changed in April and SEAD had to let go of a number of staff member and of course the pensioner was one of those to go. I felt sorry for the young ones who were paying off their cars and also renting apartments. I was not worried about losing a job at 66 years of age.

I decided to visit Pinky and her family in Canada to spend time with her husband Fintan, Hope, Aidan and latest addition to the family, Connor. I booked my ticket for June 2018 to come back in September. For the first time on all my travels I had to pay for my own ticket. R22 000 is a lot of money when you are a pensioner, fortunately, Pinky and Fin helped. I had a wonderful time with my grandchildren and thoroughly enjoyed the Canadian summer.

I came back in September to the reality of depending on my small non-governmental organisation pension. I agree with the fact that consultancy is about contacts and who you know. Very soon phone calls came requesting me to do a variety of consultation work. I have done work for United Nations Population Fund (UNFPA), the Department of Social Development, TBHIV Care. In most of the work that I am doing I depend on my skills and experience in information management, monitoring and evaluation.

There has also been a number of assignments on gender-based violence, which I find to be a challenge in the health sector. With TBHIVCare, I continued the district support in planning, monitoring and evaluation adding the Chris Hani and OR Tambo districts to Amathole. I am still continuing with TBHIVCare, supporting the HIV/AIDS/STI and TB (HAST) HAST Directorate in the department of Health.

I find retirement enjoyable. I am kept busy and learning a lot of new things especially in HIV/AIDS/TB management and also the improvements the department is making in drug supply management and distribution of treatment for chronic disease and Anti-Retroviral Treatment. I admire nurses who are at the forefront of all the changes and new regimens. They are giving the programme their all. They are also making strides in the use of computers for electronic patient information management. I am supporting all the eight districts in the province. This entails a lot of travelling and the aches and pains in my body tell me that I am 68 years old.

I recently read an article by Ted Kennan on how retirees are putting their skills to good use. It states that "One of the motivations for continuing to work after retirement is the human interaction which helps people stay young at heart and sound of mind. Consulting in particular helps one to put their knowledge, practical experience, and expertise gained in the school of life and hard knocks to good use."

I am working for my next ticket to Canada to visit Pinky, her husband Fintan, Hope Managaliso, Aidan Lizo, and Connor Rolihlahla Hartnett, my grandchildren. Your life is truly what you make it.

ABOUT THE AUTHOR

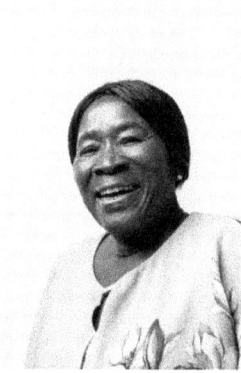

Nomathemba Mazaleni is a qualified nurse, midwife, community health nurse, nurse educator and nurse administrator. She holds a Bachelor's Degree from the University of South Africa and a Masters Degree from the University of Liverpool in the UK.

With more than 40 years in the health sector, she has worked in Public Health, Health Information System, Community Based Education for Health Personnel and HIV/ AIDS. Her extensive world travels in Asia, Europe, USA and other parts of Africa have made her the skilled professional she is.

As a health manager, leader, experienced monitoring, and evaluation practitioner, she is passionate about teaching, mentoring, supporting, and advancing the course of nurses and those who may want to follow in her footsteps.

Now in her late 60s, Nomathemba does not consider herself as Retired-only Rewired as she still works a full-time job. When not consulting professionally, she delights in being a mother and a grandmother to three lovely boys, who are the inspiration of her legacy and heritage.